Sarah Jackson

The director

Young woman's best companion

Sarah Jackson

The director
Young woman's best companion

ISBN/EAN: 9783741139826

Manufactured in Europe, USA, Canada, Australia, Japa

Cover: Foto ©Andreas Hilbeck / pixelio.de

Manufactured and distributed by brebook publishing software (www.brebook.com)

Sarah Jackson

The director

THE
DIRECTOR:
OR,

Young Woman's best Companion.

BEING

The plainest *and* cheapest *of the Kind ever published:*

The Whole makes

A Complete FAMILY COOK and PHYSICAN.

CONTAINING

Above *Three Hundred* easy RECEIPTS in

COOKERY,	CANDYING,	PHYSICK,
PASTRY,	PICKLING,	and
PRESERVING,	COLLARING,	SURGERY.

To which are added,

Plain and easy INSTRUCTIONS for choosing *Beef, Mutton, Veal, Fish, Fowl,* and other Eatables. DIRECTIONS for Carving, and to make Wines. Likewise Bills of FARE for every Month in the Year.

With a complete INDEX to the Whole.

A BOOK necessary for all Families.

By *SARAH JACKSON.*

Collected for the Use of her own Family, and printed at the Request of her Friends.

A NEW EDITION,

Corrected and greatly improved by the Author:

Particularly with an Addition of several new Cuts, which at one View shew regular and easy Forms of placing the different Sorts of Dishes from two to nine in a Course, either in the middling or genteelest Manner. With a Cut of 13 Dishes, shewing how to set off a long Table in a common Way, or after the modern Taste: Not in any other Book extant. Also several Cuts representing the trussing of Fowls, &c. Dr. *Mead's* Account of a Person bit by a mad Dog, and his infallible Cure. The Negro *Cæsar's* Cure for Poison, and likewise for the Bite of a Rattle-Snake.

LONDON:

Printed for S. CROWDER, at No. 12, and R. BALDWIN, No. 47, in *Pater-noster-Row.* 1770. [Price 1s. 6d.]

THE
PREFACE.

Addressed to Young Women in general.

AS in general young Women, when they first set out in Life, are very anxious for a Place to look after young Children, which induces me to give them some Instructions in Regard to their Behaviour in that Capacity by Way of Introduction to this little and useful Book: Then let me in the first Place advise you to consider the Charge you take in Hand, and not to desire it, as too many do, because it is an easy Kind of Life, void of Labour and Pains-taking, thinking that Children are easily pleased with any Thing; but I can assure you to the contrary, for it is a troublesome Employment, and the Charge is of greater Weight than such vainly imagine. You ought to be of a gentle and good Disposition, sober in your Carriage, neat in your Apparel; not sluggish nor heavy-headed, but watchful and careful in the Night Season, for fear any of the Children should be ill, and keep good Hours for their up-rising and going to Bed. Get their Breakfasts and Suppers in good and convenient Time, let them not sit too long, but walk them often up and down, especially those who cannot go well of themselves: Take heed they get no Falls by your Carelessness, for by such Means many (the Cause at first being unperceivable) have

PREFACE.

have afterwards grown irrecoverably lame or crooked; wherefore, if any such Thing should happen, conceal it not, though for so doing you may justly incur a great deal of Blame. Take special Care that they eat nothing which may overcharge their Stomachs. If you observe their Faces at any Time paler than ordinary, or complain of Pain in their Stomach, conclude it is the Worms that trouble them, and therefore give them Remedies suitable to the Distemper; do this often, whether you see those Symptoms or no, the Neglect of which hath been the Destruction of many hopeful Children. Keep them (whatever you do) sweet and clean, and moderately warm; and restrain them from drinking too much strong Liquors, or eating overmuch Fruit, both of which will be very prejudicial to their Health. Be not churlish or dogged to them, but merry and pleasant, and contrive or invent pretty Pastimes agreeable to their Age. Keep their Linen and other Things always mended, and suffer them not to run too fast to Decay. Do not shew a Partiality in your Love to any of them, for that dejects the rest. Be not hasty with them; have a special Care how you behave yourself before them, neither speaking nor acting misbecomingly, lest your bad Example prove the Subject of their Imitation. This is your Duty; and unless you can and will do this, never undertake this Charge. From

Your Well-wisher,

SARAH JACKSON.

THE
YOUNG WOMAN's
Best Companion.

DIRECTIONS *for* MARKETING.

How to chuse Lamb.

IN chusing a *Lamb's Head*, observe the Eyes; if they are wrinkled, or sunk in, it is stale; if lively and plump, it is new and sweet. In a *Fore-Quarter*, take notice of the Neck Vein; and if it is a Sky-Blue, it is sweet and good; but if inclining to Green or Yellow, it is almost, if not quite, tainted. In a *Hind-Quarter*, if it has a faintish Smell under the Kidney, and the Knuckle be limber, it is stale.

To chuse Mutton.

When upon pinching it between your Fingers it feels tender, and soon returns to its former Place, it is young; but if it wrinkle and remain so, it is old. If it be young, the Fat will easily separate from the Lean; but if old, it will adhere more firmly, and be very clammy and fibrous.

If it be Ram Mutton, the Fat will be spungy, the Grain close, the Lean rough and of a deep Red, and when dented with the Finger will not rise again. If the Sheep has had the Rot, the Flesh will be palish, the Fat of a faint White inclining to Yellow; the Meat will be loose at the Bone, and on your squeezing it hard, some Drops of Water, resembling a Dew or Sweat, will appear on the Surface. If it be a Fore-Quarter, observe the Vein in the Neck; for if it looks ruddy, or of an azure Colour, it is fresh; but if yellowish it is near tainting, and if green it is already tainted. As to the Hind-Quarters, smell under the Kidney, and feel whether the Knuckle be stiff or limber; for if the former has a faint or ill Scent, or the latter an unusual Limberness, you may be certain of its being stale.

To chuse Veal.

The Flesh of a Bull Calf is firmer grain'd, and redder than that of a Cow Calf, and the Fat more curled. Observe, if the Vein in the Shoulder be of a bright Red, it is new killed; but if greenish, yellowish, or blackish, or more clammy, soft, and limber than usual, it is stale; and if it hath any greenish Spots about it, it is either tainting, or already tainted. If it be wrapped in wet Cloths, it is apt to be musty; therefore always smell to it. The Loin tastes first under the Kidney, and when stale the Flesh will be soft and slimy. The Leg, if newly kill'd, will be stiff on the Joint; but if stale, limber, and the Flesh clammy, intermixed with green or yellowish Specks. The Neck and Breast are first tainted at the upper End, and when this is the Case, will have a dusky, yellowish, or greenish Appearance, and the Sweetbread on the Breast will be clammy.

To chuse Beef.

Ox Beef has an open Grain, and the Fat, if young, is of a crumbling or oily Smoothness, except it be the Brisket or Neck Pieces, with such others as are very fibrous. The Lean ought to be of a pleasant Carnation Red, the

Fat rather inclining to White than Yellow, and the Suet very white.

Cow Beef has a closer Grain, the Fat is whiter, the Bones less, and the Lean of a paler Colour. If it be young and tender, the Dent made by pressing it with the Finger will rise again in a little Time.

Bull Beef is of a deeper Red, a closer Grain, and firmer than either of the former, harder to be indented with your Finger, and rising again sooner. The Fat is gross and fibrous, and of a strong rank Scent. If it be old, it will be so very tough, that your pinching it will scarcely make any Impression. If it be fresh, it will be of a lively Colour; but if stale, of a dark dusky Colour, and very clammy. If it be bruised, the Part affected will look of a blackish or more dusky Colour than the rest.

To chuse Pork.

When upon pinching the Lean between your Fingers, it breaks and feels soft and oily, or if you can easily nip the Skin with your Nails, or if the Fat be soft and oily, it is young; but if the Lean be rough, the Fat very spungy, and the Skin stubborn, it is old. The Flesh of a Boar or Hog, gelt at full Growth, feels harder and tougher than usual, the Skin is thicker, the Fat hard and fibrous, the Lean of a dusky Red and rank Scent. That you may know it to be fresh or stale, try the Legs and Hands at the Bone which comes out in the Middle of the fleshy Part, by putting in your Finger; for as they first taint in those Places, you may easily discover it by smelling to your Finger. When stale, the Skin will be clammy and sweaty; but when fresh, it will be smooth and cool.

To chuse Brawn.

Brawn is known to be young or old by the Rind; for if it is thick and hard it is old, but if soft, and of a moderate Thickness, it is young. If the Rind and Fat be remarkably tender, it is not Boar Brawn, but Barrow or Sow.

To chuse Venison.

Before you buy a Haunch, a Shoulder, or any other fleshy Part of the Sides, take a small sharp-pointed Knife, and thrust it in where you think proper, and instantly draw it back; then apply the Blade to your Nose, which will infallibly discover whether it is rank or sweet. If you would purchase any other Part, first observe the Colour of the Meat; for, if stale, it will be blackish, and have yellowish or greenish Specks in it. If you find the Flesh tough and hard, and the Fat contracted, you may take it for granted that 'tis old.

The Season for Venison.

The *Buck* Venison begins in *May*, and is in Season till *Alhallows-Day*; the *Doe* is in Season from *Michaelmas* to the End of *December*, and sometimes to the End of *January*.

To chuse Westphalia Hams.

Try them with a small pointed Knife, as is directed above for Venison; and when you have drawn it, if you find the Blade has a fine Flavour, and is but very little daub'd, you may conclude the Ham is sweet and good; but if your Knife be all over smear'd, has a rank Scent, and a Haut-gout issue from the Vent-hole, it is certainly tainted.

To chuse English Hams and Bacon.

To chuse these, take the same Methods as with the above-mentioned Hams. In regard, however, to the other Parts, try the Fat, and if it feels oily, looks white, and does not crumble, if the Flesh bears a good Colour, and sticks close to the Bone, it is good; but if the Lean has any yellow Streaks in it, 'tis then rusty, or at least will be so in a short Time.

To chuse Butter.

When you buy Butter, do not trust to the Taste they give you, lest you be deceived by a well-tasted Piece, artfully placed in the Lump, but taste it yourself at a venture.

ture. It is easier to distinguish Salt Butter by scenting than tasting it; therefore run a Knife into it, and put it immediately to your Nose. As a Cask may be purposely pack'd, do not trust to the Top alone, but unhoop it to the Middle, and thrust down your Knife close to the Staves of the Cask, and then you cannot be deceived.

To chuse Cheese.

If the Coat of an old Cheese be rough, rugged, or dry at the Top, it indicates Mites or little Worms; or if spungy, moist, or full of Holes, it is subject to Maggots. If you perceive on the Outside any perished Place, be sure to examine its Depth.

To chuse Eggs.

When you buy Eggs hold them up against the Sun, or a Candle, and if the Whites appear clear and fair, and the Yolk round, they are good; but if muddy or cloudy, or the Yolk broken, they are naught. Or put the great End to your Tongue; if it feels warm, it is new; but if cold, it is stale. Or take the Egg and put it into a Pan of cold Water; the fresher it is, the sooner it will sink to the Bottom; but if it be rotten or addled, it will swim on the Surface of the Water. The best Way to keep them is in Bran or Meal.

To chuse Poultry.

Capons, if true, have a fat Vein on the Side of their Breasts, their Combs are pale, and their Bellies and Rumps are thick. If they are young, they have smooth Legs and short Spurs. If they are stale, their Vents are loose and open; but close and hard, if new.

To chuse a Cock or Hen.

In the Choice of a Cock, observe his Spurs; if they are short and dubbed, then he is young. If you find them either pared or scraped, you may justly be jealous of a Fraud. His Vent will be open if he be stale, but hard and close if he be new.

The Newness or Staleness of a Hen may be known by her Legs and Comb; if they are rough she is old, but if smooth she is young.

To chuse a Cock or Hen Turkey, or Turkey Poults.

If the Legs of a Turkey-Cock are black and smooth, and his Spurs short, he is young; but if his Legs are pale and rough, and his Spurs long, he is old. If long killed, his Eyes will be sunk into his Head, and his Feet feel very dry; but if fresh, his Eyes will be lively and his Feet limber. For the Hen observe the same Signs. If she be with Egg, she will have an open Vent; but if not, a close hard Vent. The same Signs will discover the Newness or Staleness of Turkey Poults.

To chuse Geese, tame or wild.

They are young if their Bills be yellowish, and they have but few Hairs; but if their Bills be red, and their Feet full of Hairs, then they are old. They are limber-footed when new, and dry-footed when stale.

To chuse Ducks, both tame and wild.

They are thick and hard on the Belly when fat, but otherwise they are lean and thin. They are limber-footed if new, and dry-footed if stale. Take notice, that the Foot of a true Wild Duck is reddish, and smaller than that of a Tame one.

To chuse Pheasants, Cocks or Hens.

The Cocks have dubbed Spurs if they be young, but in case that they are old, their Spurs will be both sharp and small. If their Vents be fast, they are new; but if they be open and flabby, then they are stale. The Hens have smooth Legs, and their Flesh is of a fine Grain, in case they are young. If they are with Egg their Vents will be open and soft, but close if they are not.

To chuse Pigeons.

The Dove-house Pigeons, when old, are red-legged; when new and fat, limber-footed, and feel full in the Vent; when stale, their Vents are green and flabby.

To chuse Hares, Leverets, and Rabbets.

When Hares are new and juſt kill'd, they will be whitiſh and ſtiff; but their Fleſh in moſt Parts will appear of a blackiſh Colour, and their Bodies will be limber, when they are ſtale. They are old when the Cleft in their Lips extends itſelf, and their Claws are wide and ragged. Obſerve the Ears well; for if they are young, they will tear with Eaſe, but be dry and tough if they be old. If you would buy a Leveret, feel on the Fore Leg, at a ſmall Bone there, you won't be impoſed on; but if you find no ſuch Thing, it is not a Leveret, but a Hare. As to Rabbets, they will be limber and ſlimy when they are ſtale, but white and ſtiff if they be new. Their Claws and Wool will be ſhort and ſmooth in caſe they be young, but long and rough if they be old.

DIRECTIONS how to chuse all Sorts of FISH.

To chuse Fresh Herrings and Mackarel.

Their Newneſs or Staleneſs is known by their keeping or loſing their lively ſhining Redneſs on their Gills; for a deadiſh fading Colour, with an ill Scent, their Fins crimpling and limber, and their Eyes looking dry and dull, ſhew that they are ſtale, whereas the contrary denotes them new.

To chuse Plaice or Flounders.

If their Eyes are any ways ſunk, or look very dull; if they are limber, and have an unuſual cold clammy Slime upon them, then are they ſtale; but if they are ſtiff, their Eyes clear and moderately dry, their Fins ſtiff, and not crimpling or ſhrivelling together, it is a Sign of Newneſs, or that they have not long been dead.

The Plaice has red or Orange-colour'd Spots on her Back, her Fins more ſpreading, of a tawnyiſh or brown Colour on the Back, has a more earthy white Belly, and her Mouth ſtanding, as it were, more awry.

The Flounder is dusky or cloudy on the Back, without Spots, thicker and more compact, and has a kind of an azurish white Belly.

To chuse Maids and Thornbacks.

The Staleness appears in these by their Eyes beginning to sink and look dull, their Flesh feeling flabby, their Lips beginning to hang, and the Corners of their Mouths to be corrupted: But when no such bad Signs appear, they may well enough pass for new.

To chuse Turbots, Cod, Fresh Salmon, Carp, Pike, Bream, Roach, Trout, Grayling, Ruff, Chub, Tench, Eel, Barbel, Whiting, Smelts, &c.

These, and all such-like Fish, if new, will be stiff, and their Eyes well standing and of a lively Colour; but when they begin to taint, their cold slimy Substance makes them limber; the Moisture falling from the Brain renders the Eyes more dull, and, as it were, shrinking or sinking; their Fins, though often wetted by the Fishmongers to prevent it, will however crimple, and shew Signs of approaching Putrefaction.

To chuse Pickled Salmon.

If the Scales are bright and shining, of a light azure Colour, the Skin, when press'd down, rising again quickly, the Flesh of a blushing Colour, and of a pleasant Scent, then it is good: But if the Scales are cloudy, dark, easily slip off the Skin, rough and stubborn, the Flakes short, dry and brittle, then is the Goodness gone from it, and it is either decay'd Fish, or has been recovered by Pickle after Damage.

To chuse Lobsters.

The Cock is usually smaller than the Hen, and of a deeper Red when boiled; neither has it any Spawn or Seed under its Tail.

To know whether these are new or stale, unbend the Tail, and if it be stiff in opening, and snap to again, then it is new; but if limber and flagging, it is stale. If new, it has a pleasant Scent at that Part of the Tail which joins to the Body; if it is spent, a white Scurf will issue out of the Roots of the small Legs, and at the Mouth. To see whether it is full, open it with the Point of a Knife on the Bend of the Tail, as it is tied down; and if it fill the Shell there, and be red, hard, and pleasant scented, it is good; but if sinking and soft, it is spent and wasted; for the Fishmonger, to deceive the ignorant Buyer, will only open them at the extreme Part of the Tail; and tho' they be wasted, they will appear well enough there. If you suspect the Claws filled with Water to make them weighty, as sometimes they do, pull out a Plug you will find there, and the Water will gush out.

To chuse Crab-Fish great and small.

If stale, the Joints of their Claws will be limber, the Colour of their Shells of a dusky Red, and an ill Scent just under the Throat; their Eyes will be very loose, turn any way with the Tip of your Finger, and sink inward.

To chuse Scate.

Chuse them by their Thickness; and the She-Scate is always the sweetest, especially if large.

To chuse Prawns and Shrimps.

If new, they will be hard and stiff, cast a pleasant Scent, and their Tails turn strongly inward: But if stale, they will be limber, and fade in their Colour, smell faintly, and feel clammy.

To chuse Cod and Codlings.

Such are best that are thick towards the Head, and whose Flesh when cut is perfectly white.

To chuse Sturgeon.

If it cuts without crumbling, and the Veins and Gristle give a true Blue where they appear, and the Flesh a perfect White, then conclude it to be good.

Salt Cod and Old Ling

Are known to be good when the Flakes rise well and oily, the Bone parts clean from the Flesh, and they are of a bright natural Colour, and good Scent; but they are bad when they break short, are hard and dry, change Colour, the Skin rough, sticking close, not well to be stirred or removed.

To chuse Pickled Herrings and Pilchards.

Open the Back; if the Flesh be soft and mellow, kindly parting from the Bone, comes out in long Flakes, the Bone white, and somewhat inclining to a light Red, then are they new and good; but if the Flesh stick to the Bone, be brittle and rough, the Bone of a yellowish, blackish, or murrey Colour, they are rusty, and of little Worth.

To chuse Red Herrings.

If they carry a good Gloss, and the Flesh part kindly from the Bone, and they be of a light bright Colour, they are good; but the contrary shews them decay'd or rusty.

To chuse Anchovies.

Open the Cork in the Middle of the Head of the Barrel, put in your Little Finger, and taste the Pickle: If it tastes mellow, has a good Relish, and looks of a dusky Red, then it is the natural Pickle, and they may prove well; but if it be whitish, watry, rough, and very brackish, it signifies new Pickle has been put to them. But to try the Fish, open the Backs of two or three of them; and if the Flesh be of a pleasant Red, soft and mellow, the Bone moist and oily, the Flesh easily parting to good Lengths without breaking, then are they good; but if it be stiff, brittle, of a dusky Colour, the Bone dry, and of a whitish Yellow, or blackish, then they are decay'd, or have been rusty, and artificially recovered, and consequently naught.

BREAD.

BREAD.

I think it not improper to give our Readers the Weight and Sizes of the different Loaves, made by the Authority of the Magistrates. A Peck Loaf to weigh 17 Pounds, 6 Ounces, 1 Dram; a Half-Peck Loaf to weigh 8 Pounds, 11 Ounces, and half a Dram; a Quartern Loaf to weigh 4 Pounds, 5 Ounces, 8 Drams and a Quarter.

The proper Seasons of all Sorts of Provisions.

House-Lamb is in its high Season particularly at *Christmas*, though it is to be procured all the Year round.

Grass-Lamb begins to be in Season in *April*, and holds good to the Middle of *August*.

Mutton, Veal, and Beef, are in Season all the Year.

Pig and Pork come in Season at *Bartholomew-Tide*, and hold good till *Lady-Day*.

Poultry in Season.

January: Turkeys, Capons, Pullets, Fowls, Chickens, Hares, all Sorts of Wild Fowl, Tame Rabbits, and Tame Pigeons.

February The same as *January*, with Green Geese, Ducklings, and Turkey-Poults. *Note*, In this Month all Sorts of Wild Fowl begin to decay.

March: This Month the same as the last; with this Difference only, that Wild Fowl are now quite out of Season.

April: Pullets, Fowls, Chickens, Pigeons, young Wild Rabbits, Leverets, young Geese, Ducklings, and Turkey-Poults.

May, June, July: The same; only add to this last, Partridges, Pheasants, and Wild Ducks.

August: The same.

September, October, November, December: All Sorts of Fowls, both Wild and Tame; but particularly Wild Fowl are in high Season the three Months last above mentioned.

Fish in Season.

From *Lady-Day* to *Midsummer*, Lobsters, **Crabs**, Crayfish, Mackarel, Breams, Barbel, Roach, Shad, Lampreys or Lamper Eels and Dace. Note as to Eels, such as are catched in running Water are looked upon as preferable to any Pond Eels, but for these last the Silver ones are in most Esteem.

From *Midsummer* to *Michaelmas*, Turbot, Trout, **Soals**, Grigs, Salmon, Sturgeon, Lobsters, and Crabs.

From *Michaelmas* to *Christmas*, Cod and Haddock, Ling, Herrings, Sprats, Soals, Flounders, Plaice, Dabs, Eels, Chare, Thornbacks, Oysters, Salmon, Perch, Carp, Pike, and Tench.

In this Quarter, Smelts are in high Season, and hold till after *Christmas*.

From *Christmas* to *Lady-Day*, Gudgeons, **Smelts**, Perch, Anchovy and Loach, Scollops, Periwincles, Cockles, and Muscles.

INSTRUCTIONS *for* DRESSING *all Sorts of* Common Provisions.

Rules for Roasting.

Make your Fire in the first place in Proportion to the Joint you dress (be it what it will) but whether small or large, let it be clear and brisk. If your Joint be larger than ordinary, take care to lay a good Fire to cake; and keep it always clear from Ashes at the Bottom.

When you imagine your Meat half done, move the Spit and Dripping-Pan at some small Distance from the Fire, which you must then stir up, and make it burn as brisk as you can; for observe, the quicker your Fire, the better and more expeditiously will your Meat be roasted.

To roast a Rib of Beef.

For the first half Hour sprinkle your Meat with Salt, then dry and flour it; after that, take a large Piece of Paper and butter it well, when you have so done, fasten it on the Butter Side to the Meat, and then let it remain till your Meat is enough.

To roast a Rump or Surloin of Beef.

Don't salt either of them in the Manner you do your Ribs; but lay them at a convenient Distance from the Fire, then baste them once or twice with Salt and Water, but afterwards with Butter; then flour them, and keep constantly basting them with what drops from them.

To make Gravy for Roast Beef.

Take three Spoonfuls of Vinegar, about a Pint of boiling Water, a Shallot or two, and a small Piece of Horseradish, add to these two Spoonfuls of Catchup, and one Glass of Claret. When your Meat is near done, put these Ingredients into a clean Dish under your Meat while it is roasting, baste it with this two or three Times; then strain it and put it under your Meat: Garnish your Dish with Horse-radish and red Cabbage.

To roast Mutton and Lamb.

Make your Fire quick and clear before you lay your Meat down, baste it often whilst it is roasting, and when almost enough, dredge it with a small Quantity of Flour.

N. B. If it be a Breast, remember to take off the Skin before you lay it down.

To roast Veal.

If it be a Shoulder, baste it with Milk till it is near half done, then flour it and baste it with Butter; if you intend to stuff it, take the same Materials as you would for a Fillet.

The Ingredients for a Fillet are these that follow: Take what Quantity you think proper of Thyme, Marjoram, Parsley, a small Onion, a Sprig of Savory, a small Quantity of Lemon-peel cut very fine, Nutmeg, Pepper, Mace,

Crumbs of Bread, three or four Eggs, a Quarter of a Pound of Marrow or Butter, with Flour intermixed in order to make it stiff. Put one Half of your Stuffing thus prepared into the Udder, and distribute the Remainder in such a Number of Holes as you think convenient to make in the fleshy Part.

If you have the Loin to roast, cover it over with a clean Piece of Paper, that as little of the Kidney Fat may be lost as possible. If it be a Breast, it must be covered with the Caul, and the Sweetbread must be fastened with a Skewer on the Backside; when it is near enough take the Caul off, then baste it and dredge it well with Flour.

Serve it up with a proper Quantity of melted Butter, and let your Dish be garnished with Lemon.

To roast Pork.

When your Pork is laid down, let it be some Distance from the Fire for a while, and take care to flour it pretty thick; when you find the Flour begins to dry, wipe it perfectly clean with a coarse Cloth; then take a sharp Knife, if it be a Loin, and cut the Skin across; after you have so done, raise your Fire, and put your Meat nearer to it than before; baste it well, and roast it as quick as you can.

If it be a Leg, you must make your Incisions very deep, when it is almost ready, fill up the Cuts with grated Bread, Sage, Parsley, a small Quantity of Lemon-peel cut fine, a Bit of Butter, about two or three Eggs, and a little Pepper, Salt, and Nutmeg mixed together: When it is full enough, serve it up with Gravy and Apple-sauce.

If you intend to roast a Spare-rib, you must baste it with Butter, Flour, and Sage shred very small: When enough, send it to Table with a proper Quantity of Apple-sauce.

If Pork is not well done, it is apt to surfeit.

To roast a Pig.

Before you put your Pig on the Spit, let it lie for a Quarter of an Hour in warm Milk, then take it out and wipe

wipe it perfectly dry; then take a Quarter of a Pound of Butter, and about the same Weight in Crumbs of Bread, a small Quantity of Sage, Thyme, Parsley, Sweet Marjoram, Pepper, Salt, and Nutmeg, and the Yolks of two or three Eggs; mingle these all well together, and sew it up in the Belly: After this flour it very thick, and then put it on the Spit; and when you lay it to the Fire, take care that both Ends of it burn clear, or else hang a flat Iron on the Middle of the Grate till you find they do. When the Crackling begins to grow hard, wipe it clean with a Cloth that has been purposely wetted in Salt and Water, then baste it well with Butter. As soon as you find the Gravy begins to run, put a Bason or two into the Dripping-pan to catch what falls: When your Pig is enough, take about a Quarter of a Pound of Butter and put it into a coarse Cloth, and after you have made your Fire perfectly clear and brisk, rub your Pig with it all over, till the Crackling is quite crisp, and then take it from the Fire. Before you take it from the Spit, cut the Head off first, and then the Body into two Parts; after that cut the Ears off, and place one at each End; as also divide the under Jaw in two, and place one Part on each Side. When Matters are thus far prepared melt some Butter, mix it with the Gravy, the Brains when bruised, and a small Quantity of Sage shred small; and then serve it up to Table.

To roast a Hare with a Pudding in his Belly.

When you have washed the Hare, nick the Legs through the Joints, and skewer them on both Sides, which will keep it from drying in the Roasting; when you have skewer'd her, put the Pudding into her Belly, baste it with nothing but Butter, put a little in the Dripping-pan: When your Hare is enough, take the Gravey out of the Dripping-pan, and thicken it up with a little Flour and Butter for the Sauce.

To make a Pudding for a Hare.

Take the Liver, a little Beef Suet, Sweet Marjoram and

and Parsley shred small, with Bread Crumbs and two Eggs; season it with Nutmeg, Pepper, and Salt, to your Taste, mix all together, and if it be too stiff, put in a Spoonful or two of Cream. You must not boil the Liver.

To roast Rabbets.

When they are laid down, baste them well with good Butter, and then dredge them with Flour if they be young and small; let your Fire be clear: They will be enough in about Half an Hour, but if they are large, give them a Quarter of an Hour's roasting longer. Before you take them up, melt a proper Quantity of good Butter; and when you have boiled their Livers with a Bunch of Parsley and shred them small, put one Half into your Butter, and pour it under them, and reserve the rest to garnish your Dish.

To roast Pigeons.

Take some Parsley and cut it small, then take a little Pepper, Salt, and a small Piece of Butter, mix these all together, and put them into the Bellies of your Pigeons, tying the Neck Ends tight, fasten one End of another String to their Legs and Rumps, and the other to your Mantle-piece. Keep them constantly turning round, and baste them well with Butter; when enough, serve them up, and they'll swim with Gravy.

To roast Venison.

In the first place prepare some Vinegar and Water to wash your Venison in, and dry it afterwards with a clean Cloth, then either cover it with the Caul, or with Paper very plentifully buttered; lay it down before a clear Fire and keep basting it with Butter till it is almost enough; after this, take a Pint of Claret, put some whole Pepper, Nutmeg, Cloves, and Mace to it, and boil them all together in a Sauce-pan; pour this Liquor twice over your Venison; after that, take it up, and after you have strained it, serve it up in the same Dish as your Venison, then place a sufficient Quantity of Gravy on one Side of your Dish and sweet Sauce on the other.

To roast Mutton, Venison Fashion.

Take a hind Quarter of Mutton that is fat, and cut the Leg as you would a Haunch of Venison, then rub it well with a proper Quantity of Salt-petre, and hang it up for two or three Days in some moist Place; but wipe it, however, with a clean Cloth, at least twice a Day: After this, put it into a Pan, then boil a Quarter of an Ounce of All Spice in a Quart of Claret, and pour it boiling-hot into your Pan, then let it stand covered for two or three Hours. Thus prepared, it is ready for the Spit; lay it to the Fire, and constantly basting it with Butter and some of your Liquor, it will be ready in an Hour and a Half, if your Fire be clear, and your Joint be of a moderate Bigness. When taken up, send it to Table with a proper Quantity of Gravy in one Bason, and some sweet Sauce in the other.

To roast a Goose.

Take a little Sage, and a small Onion chopt small, some Pepper and Salt, and a Bit of Butter, mix these together, and put into the Belly of the Goose. Then spit it, singe it with a Bit of white Paper, dredge it with a little Flour, and baste it with Butter. When it is done, which may be known by the Legs being tender, take it up, and pour through it two Glasses of red Wine, and serve it up in the same Dish, and some Apple-sauce in a Bason.

To roast a Turkey.

Before you lay it down, take about a Quarter of a Pound of lean Veal, a small Quantity of Thyme, Parsley, Sweet Marjoram, some Winter Savory, a small Quantity of Lemon-peel, and one Onion shred small; add to these, a grated Nutmeg, a small Quantity of Salt, a Dram of Mace, and Half a Pound of Butter; pound your Meat as small as possible, and cut your Herbs likewise very small; when your Materials are thus prepared, mix them all together with two or three Eggs, and as much Flour or Crumbs of Bread as will make the Whole of a proper Confiſtence: Fill the Crop of your Turkey with the ſavory Ingredients; after that, lay it down at a ſmall Diſtance from the Fire. In about an Hour and a Quarter it will be enough, if it be of a moderate Size; but if very large, allow it a Quarter of an Hour longer.

To roaſt the hind Quarter of a Pig, Lamb Faſhion.

At the Time of Year when Houſe-Lamb is very dear, take the hind Quarter of a large Pig, take off the Skin, and roaſt it, and it will eat like Lamb, with Mint Sauce, or with a Sallad, or *Seville* Oranges.

To roaſt a Leg of Mutton with Cockles or Oyſters.

Take a Leg about two or three Days old, ſtuff it all over with Cockles or Oyſters and roaſt it; garniſh your Diſh with Horſe-radiſh.

To roaſt a Tongue or Udder.

Parboil your Tongue or Udder, then ſtick into it ten or twelve Cloves, and whilſt it is roaſting baſte it with Butter; when it is ready, take it up and ſend it to Table with ſome Gravy and ſweet Sauce.

To roaſt a Calf's Liver.

Lard your Liver well with large Slices of Bacon, faſten it on a Spit, roaſt it at a gentle Fire, and ſerve it up with good Veal Gravy, or a Poivrade.

A good Sauce for Teal, Mallard, Ducks, &c.

Take a Quantity of Veal Gravy, according to the Bigneſs of your Diſh of Wild Fowl, ſeaſoned with Pepper and Salt, ſqueeze in the Juice of two Oranges, and a little Claret; this will ſerve all Sorts of Wild Fowl.

Directions *concerning* Poultry.

If your Fire is not very quick and clear when you lay your Poultry down to roaſt, it will not eat ſo ſweet or look ſo beautiful to the Eye.

To roast an Eel.

Take a great Eel, flit the Skin a little Way, then pull off the Skin, Head and all, parboil the Eel till it comes from the Bone, then shred it with some Oysters, sweet Herbs, and Lemon-peel, season it with Salt; scower the Skin with Salt and Water, and stuff it full again with the Meat, sew it up and roast it with Butter; for Sauce, take some white Wine, dissolve three Anchovies in it, and beat as much Butter as will serve for Sauce; then serve it up.

To dress Rabbets like Moor Game.

Take a young Rabbet, when it is cased, cut off the Wings and the Head; leave the Neck of your Rabbet as long as you can; when you case it you must leave on the Feet and Claws, and pull off the Skin, then double your Rabbet and skewer it like a Fowl; put a Skewer at the Bottom through the Legs and Neck, and tie it with a String, it will prevent it flying open. When you dish it up make the same Sauce as you would do for Partridges. Three is enough for one Dish.

To roast Woodcocks and Snipes.

Put them on a little Spit proper for the Purpose, toast Part of a Three-penny Loaf brown, and put it in a Dish, which you must set under your Birds; baste them well with Butter, and let the Trail drop on the Toast at the Bottom of your Dish, and your Birds. Take care to have Half a Pint of good Gravy ready to pour into a Dish; and serve them up.

N. B. Never take any Thing out of a Woodcock or Snipe; nor ever put any Ingredients into the Bellies of your Wild Ducks, as you do either into Tame ones or into Geese.

To roast Larks.

Truss them handsomely on the Back, but neither draw them nor cut off their Feet: Lard them with small Lardoons, or else spit them on a wooden Skewer, with a small Lard of Bacon between two; when they are near roasted enough,

enough, dredge them with Salt powdered fine, and fine Crumbs of Bread. When they are ready, rub the Dish you defign to ferve them in with a Shalot, and ferve them with Salt and Pepper, Verjuice, and the Juice of an Orange and Crumbs of Bread fried, and ferve them in a Plate by themfelves; or with a Sauce made of Claret, the Juice of two or three Oranges, and a little fhred Ginger, fet over the Fire a little while with a Bit of Butter. You may ufe the fame Sauce for broiled Larks, which you muft open on the Breafts when you lay them upon the Gridiron.

General Directions for Boiling.

KNOW the Weight of your Meat before you put it into your Pot; be your Joint fmall or large, allow a Quarter of an Hour for every Pound; take care before you put your Meat in, that your Pot be perfectly neat and clean, as well as the Water that you put in. When your Water begins to fimmer fkim it well, for a Skum will always rife; and if through Carelefnefs you let it boil down, your Meat will be black, or of a dingy Colour.

N. B. You muft put all Meats that are well falted into your Water whilft it is cold. But your Water muft boil firft before you put in your frefh Meats, of what Nature or Kind foever.

To boil a Leg of Lamb, with the Loin fry'd.

When your Lamb is boiled lay it in the Difh, and pour upon it a little Parfley, Butter, and green Goofeberries coddled, then lay your fried Lamb round it; take fome fmall Afparagus, and cut it fmall like Peafe, and boil it green, when it is boiled drain it in a Cullinder, and lay it round your Lamb in Spoonfuls. Garnifh your Difh with Goofeberries, and Heads of Afparagus in Lumps. This is proper for a Bottom Difh.

To boil a Leg of Lamb with Chickens.

When your Lamb is boiled pour over it Parſley and Butter, with coddled Gooſeberries; lay your Chickens round your Lamb, and pour over the Chickens a little white Fricaſſee Sauce. Garniſh your Diſh with Sippets and Lemon. This is proper for a Top Diſh.

To boil a Ham.

Put your Ham into a Copper in Caſe you have one, let it lie there for three or four Hours ſucceſſively before you let your Water boil, but keep ſcumming it all the Time notwithſtanding; after that, make your Copper boil, and then, in an Hour and a Half it will be enough in caſe it is but ſmall; and two Hours will be ſufficient if it be large.

To boil a Tongue.

If your Tongue be ſalt, put it into your Pot over Night, but don't let it boil till about three Hours before you intend to ſerve it up to Table. Take care that it boils all thoſe three Hours; if freſh out of the Pickle, two Hours; but let your Water boil before you put it in.

To boil pickled Pork.

Waſh your Pork and ſcrape it clean, then put it in when the Water is cold, and let it boil till the Rind be tender.

To boil a Duck or Rabbet with Onions.

Let your Rabbet or Duck be boiled in Plenty of Water, and as a Scum will always riſe, be ſure to take it off, for if it boils down, it will either blacken or diſcolour, at leaſt, your Meat: Give them about Half an Hour's boiling. As for your Sauce, firſt peel your Onions, and as you peel them throw them into cold Water, then take them out, and cut them into Slices; boil them in Milk and Water, and ſkim the Liquor. They will not require above Half an Hour's boiling; when they are enough, throw them into a clean Sieve in order to drain them; then, when you have chopt them ſmall, put them into a Sauce-

Sauce-pan, duſt them with a little Flour, put two or three Spoonfuls of Cream to them, a large Bit of Butter, ſtew them over the Fire all together, and when they are fine or thick, lay your Duck or Rabbet into your Diſh, and bury it as it were with your Sauce. If it be a Rabbet cut the Head in two, and lay the Parts ſo divided on each Side of the Diſh. If it be a Duck for Change make the following Sauce; cut an Onion ſmall, then take half a Handful of Parſley clean pick'd and well waſhed, let it be chopt ſmall; cut a Lettuce likewiſe ſmall; then take about a Quarter of a Pint of good Gravy, and a Lump of Butter rolled in Flour; ſqueeze ſome Lemon Juice into it, and add a little Pepper and Salt; ſtew theſe all together for about Half and Hour, then enrich it with two or three Spoonfuls of red Wine.

To boil a Gooſe.

When your Gooſe has been ſeaſoned with Pepper and Salt for four or five Days, you muſt boil it about an Hour; then ſerve it hot with Turnips, Carrots, Cabbage, or Collyflowers, toſſed up with Butter.

To boil Pigeons.

Let your Pigeons be boiled by themſelves for about a Quarter of an Hour; then boil a proper Quantity of Bacon cut ſquare, and lay it in the Middle of your Diſh. Stew ſome Spinage; garniſh with Parſley dried criſp before the Fire.

To boil Pheaſants.

Let them have a good deal of Water, and keep it boiling; Half an Hour will be ſufficient for ſmall ones, but allow three Quarters if your Pheaſants are large. Let your Sauce conſiſt of Sellery ſtewed with Cream; add to it a ſmall Lump of Butter rolled in Flour: When you have taken them up, pour your Sauce all over them. Garniſh your Diſh with Lemon.

To boil Rabbets.

Truſs them and boil them white and quick: For Sauce, boil and ſhred the Livers, and ſome Parſley ſhred fine; add

to

to them some Capers, and mingle all these with about Half a Pint of Gravy, a Glass of white Wine, a little Mace, Nutmeg, Pepper and Salt, and a Lump of Butter about the Bigness of a Walnut rolled in Flour; let it all boil together till it is thick, then take up your Rabbets, and pour your Sauce over them. Garnish your Dish with Lemon.

To boil Chickens.

Take four or five Chickens, as you would have your Dish in Bigness; if they be small ones scald them before you pluck them, and take out the Breast-bone; wash them, truss them, cut off their Heads and Necks, and boil them in Milk and Water, with a little Salt: Half an Hour or less will boil them. They are better for being killed the Night before you use them.

To make Sauce for Chickens.

Take the Necks, Gizzards, and Livers, boil them in Water; when they are enough strain off the Gravy, and put to it a Spoonful of Oyster-pickle: Take the Livers, break them small, mix with them a little Gravy, and rub them through a Hair Sieve with the Back of a Spoon; then put to it a Spoonful of Cream, a little Lemon, and Lemon-peel grated; thicken it up with Butter and Flour Let your Sauce be no thicker than Cream, which pour upon your Chickens. Garnish your Dish with Sippets, Mushrooms, and Slices of Lemon. They are proper for a Side-Dish or Top-Dish, either at Noon or Night.

To boil a Turkey.

When your Turkey is dressed and drawn, truss it, cut off his Feet, take down the Breast-bone with a Knife, and sew up the Skin again; stuff the Breast with a white Stuffing.

To make the Stuffing.

Take the Sweetbread of a Calf, boil it, shred it fine, with a little Beef-suet, a Handful of Bread-crumbs, a little Lemon-peel, Part of a Liver, a Spoonful or two of Cream,

Cream, with Nutmeg, Pepper, Salt, and two Eggs, mix all together, and stuff your Turkey with Part of the Stuffing, (the rest you may either boil or fry to lay round it) dredge it with a little Flour, tie it up in a Cloth, and boil it with Milk and Water. If it be a young Turkey an Hour will boil it.

To make Sauce for a Turkey.

Take a little small white Gravy, a Pint of Oysters, two or three Spoonfuls of Cream, a little Juice of Lemon, and Salt to your Taste; thicken it up with Flour and Butter, then pour it over the Turkey, and serve it up; lay round your Turkey fried Oysters and Forced-Meat. Garnish your Dish with Oysters, Mushrooms, and Slices of Lemon.

To make another Sauce for a Turkey.

Take a little strong white Gravy, with some of the whitest Sellery you can get, cut it about an Inch long, boil it till it be tender, and put it into the Gravy, with two Anchovies, a little Lemon-peel shred, two or three Spoonfuls of Cream, a little Mace shred, and a Spoonful of white Wine; thicken it up with Flour and Butter. If you dislike the Sellery, you may put in the Liver as you did for Chickens.

Instructions with Regard to Greens, Roots, and other Produce of the Kitchen-Garden.

MOST injudicious Cook-maids, for the Generality, spoil all their Materials from the Garden by boiling them over-much. All Greens of what Denomination soever should have a Crispness, for in Case they happen to be over-boiled, not only their Beauty, but their Sweetness too, is lost.

Before

Before you put your Greens, however, into your Pot, take particular Care to pick them, and wash them well. For fear of any Dust or Sand, which is too apt to hang round wooden Vessels, lay them always in a clean earthen Pan. Let your Greens be boiled in a large Quantity of Water, and in a Copper Saucepan by themselves; for whenever you boil them with your Meat, you will always find that they will be discoloured. Take notice, that no Iron Pans are proper for this Purpose; always make use, therefore, of Copper or Brass.

To dress Carrots.

In the first place, scrape them very clean, and rub them well with a coarse Cloth as soon as you find them enough. After that, slide them into a Plate, and pour over them a proper Quantity of melted Butter. They will not require above half an Hour's boiling in case they be young Carrots; if they are large, they will require twice that Time; but if they be your old *Sandwich* Carrots, you must give them two Hours boiling at least.

To boil Cabbage or Savoy Sprouts.

If your Savoys be cabbaged, dress off the out Leaves, and cut them in Quarters; take off a little of the hard Ends, and boil them in a large Quantity of Water with a little Salt; when boiled drain them, lay them round your Meat, and pour over them a little Butter. Any thing will boil greener in a large Quantity of Water than otherwise.

To dress Spinage.

Let it, in the first place, be pick'd very clean, and then wash'd in several Waters; put it into a Saucepan that will but just boil it, and when you have strewed a small Quantity of Salt over it, cover up your Pan, shake it often, but put no Water to it. Let your Fire be clear and quick, over which you set your Saucepan. When you find that your Greens are shrunk to the Bottom, and the Liquor proceeding from them boils up, take them up, and throw them into a clean Sieve, and drain them well, by giving them a Squeeze or two; then lay them in a clean Plate, but put no Butter over them. Have a small Bason, however, ready, and set it in the Middle for every body at Table to take what Quantity they think best.

Spinage with poach'd Eggs is a Dish very much used at Supper.

To boil Broccoli.

Take Broccoli when it is seeded, or at any other Time; take off all the low Leaves from your Stalks, and tie them up in Bunches as you do Asparagus; cut them in little Pieces, of the same Length you peel your Stalks. You must let your Water boil before you put them in. Boil your Heads in Salt and Water, and let the Water boil before you put in the Broccoli; put in a little Butter. It takes very little boiling, and if it boils too quick it will take off all the Heads. You must drain your Broccoli through a Sieve, as you do Asparagus. Lay the Stalks in the Middle, and the Bunches round them, as you would do Asparagus.

This is proper either for a Side-dish or a Middle-dish.

To boil Asparagus.

Be careful to scrape all your Stalks till they look white; then cut them all even, and tie them up in small Bundles. Have your Stew-pan ready with boiling Water, and throw them into it, together with some Salt. Keep your Water constantly boiling, and take them up when you find them tender. They will not only lose their Colour, but their Taste likewise, if you let them boil too much. Cut the Round of a small Loaf, about half an Inch thick; toast it well on both Sides, dip it in your Asparagus Liquor, and lay it in your Dish; then pour some melted Butter over your Toast, and lay your Asparagus upon it, and all round the Dish, with the white Tops towards the

Edge

Edge of the Dish. Pour no Butter over your Asparagus, but have some melted to serve up with it in a Bason

To boil Turnips.

Boil these in the Pot with your Meat, for they eat best so. When they are enough, put them into a Pan, and mash them with a large Lump of Butter, and a small Quantity of Salt. Some good Cooks pare them, and cut them into Pieces; then put them into a clean Saucepan, with Water just enough. When boil'd, they drain them through a Sieve, then put them into a Saucepan with a good Lump of Butter, and after they have kept stirring them over the Fire a few Minutes, serve them up to Table. Others again take them up whole, and after squeezing them between two Trenchers, to drain the Liquor from them, pour melted Butter over them, and serve them up.

To boil Potatoes.

Boil them with no more Water than what will just save your Saucepan from burning. Let your Saucepan be cover'd close, and when they are enough their Skin will begin to crack. Let all the Water that you find in them be first well drain'd out, and then cover them again for about two or three Minutes; after this peel them, and lay them in a Plate; then pour melted Butter over them. Your best Cooks, however, when they have peel'd them, put them on a Gridiron, and let them lie till they are of a fine Brown, and so serve them up. Others again put them into a Saucepan with some good Beef Dripping, and cover them close, shake them often, and when they are crisp, and of a fine Brown, take them up in a Plate; but for fear of any Fat, remove them into another, and then serve them up, with a small Bason of melted Butter.

To boil Parsnips.

Let them be boiled in Plenty of Water; and when, by running your Fork into them, you find they are soft, take them up, and scrape them perfectly clean, but throw away the thick Parts: Then have a Saucepan ready with some Milk in it, and throw them into it; but keep ſtirring them over the Fire till they are of a proper Confiſtence. Don't let them burn, but put a good Lump of Butter to them, and ſome Salt. When your Butter is perfectly melted, ſerve them up.

To boil Artichokes.

When you have wrung their Stalks off, put them into cold Water with their Tops downwards, by which means all the Duſt and Sand that are in them will boil out. When the Water once boils, they will be ready in about an Hour and a half. Serve them up with melted Butter in little Cups.

To boil French Beans.

String them in the firſt place, then cut them in two, and after that acroſs; or, which is a nicer Way, cut them in four, and then acroſs, which makes eight Pieces. Lay them in Water and Salt, and when your Pan boils, throw in firſt a ſmall Quantity of Salt, and afterwards your Beans into the Water. They are enough as ſoon as they are tender. Take as much Care as you can to preſerve their lively Green; lay them in a ſmall Diſh, and ſerve them up with a Baſon of melted Butter.

To boil Cauliflowers.

Cut off all the green Part of your Flowers, and then cut your Flowers into four Parts. Let them lie in Water for an Hour: Then have ſome Milk and Water boiling; put your Flowers in, and ſkim your Saucepan well. As ſoon as you find the Stalks tender, take them up, and carefully put them into a Cullender to drain. Then put a Spoonful or two of Water into a clean Stewpan, with a little Duſt of Flour, and about a Quartern of Butter; ſhake it round till well melted, together with a little Pepper and Salt. Then take half the Cauliflower, and cut it in the ſame Manner as if you were to pickle it, and lay it in your Stewpan; turn it, and ſhake the Pan round;

it

it will be enough in ten Minutes. Lay the stew'd Part of your Flowers into the Middle of a small Dish, and the boil'd round it; pour the Butter you did it in over, and serve it up.

How to keep Meat hot.

The best Way to keep Meat hot, if it be done before your Company is ready, is to set the Dish over a Pan of boiling Water; cover your Dish with a deep Cover, so as not to touch the Meat, and throw a Cloth over all. Thus you may keep your Meat hot a long time, and it is better than over-roasting and spoiling it. The Steam of the Water keeps the Meat hot, and does not draw the Gravy out, or dry it up; whereas if you set a Dish of Meat any Time over a Chafing-dish of Coals, it will dry up the Gravy, and spoil the Meat.

INSTRUCTIONS *for dressing all Sorts of* FISH.

To broil Herrings and Sprats.

LET your Fire be very brisk, and your Gridiron hot; then wipe them dry with a coarse Cloth, flour them well, and chalk your Gridiron. Keep them constantly turning; and when their Flesh parts from the Bone, they are enough. Melt some Butter with Mustard, and serve them up to Table.

To fry Herrings.

Scale and wash your Herrings clean, strew over them a little Flour and Salt; let your Butter be very hot before put your Herrings into the Pan; then shake it to keep them stirring, and fry them over a brisk Fire. When they are fried cut off their Heads and bruise them; put to them a Gill of Ale, (but the Ale must not be bitter) add a little Pepper and Salt, a small Onion or Shalot if you have them, and boil them all together. When they are boiled, strain them, and put them into your Saucepan again;

thicken

thicken them with a little Flour and Butter, put it into a Bason, and set it in the Middle of your Dish; fry the Milts and Roes together, and lay round your Herrings. Garnish your Dish with crisp Parsley, and serve it up.

To boil Herrings.

Take your Herrings, scale, and wash them; take out the Milt and Roe, skewer them round, and tie them in a String, or else they will come loose in the boiling, and be spoiled. Set on a pretty broad Stewpan, with as much Water as will cover them; put to it a little Salt, and lay in your Herrings with the Backs downwards; boil with them the Milts and Roes, to lie round them; they will boil in half a Quarter of an Hour over a slow Fire. When they are boiled, take them up with an Egg-Slice to turn them over, and set them to drain. Make your Sauce of a little Gravy and Butter, an Anchovy, and a little boiled Parsley shred; put it into a Bason, set it in the Middle of the Dish; lay the Herrings round, with their Tails towards the Bason, and lay the Milts and Roes betwixt every Herring. Garnish with crisp Parsley and Lemon; so serve them up.

To pickle Herrings.

Scale and clean your Herrings, take out the Milts and Roes, and skewer them round; season them with a little Pepper and Salt, put them in a deep Pot, cover them with Alegar, put to them a little whole *Jamaica* Pepper, and two or three Bay-leaves; bake them, and keep them for Use.

To keep Herrings all the Year.

Take fresh Herrings, cut off their Heads, open and wash them very clean, season them with Salt, black Pepper, and *Jamaica* Pepper; put them into a Pot, cover them with White-wine Vinegar and Water, of each an equal Quantity, and set them in a slow Oven to bake; tie the Pot up close, and they will keep a Year in the Pickle.

To broil Whitings.

Whitings should be washed with Water and Salt, then dry them well, and flour them; rub your Gridiron well with Chalk, and make it hot; then lay on, and when they are enough, serve them with Oyster or Shrimp Sauce: Garnish them with Lemon sliced. *N. B.* The Chalk will keep the Fish from sticking.

To dress a Cod's Head.

Take a Cod's Head, wash and clean it; take out the Gills, cut it open, and make it to lie flat. If you have not Conveniency of boiling it, you may do it in an Oven, and it will be as well or better. Put it into a Copper Dish, or an earthen one, lay upon it a little Butter, Salt, and Flour, and when it is enough take off the Skin.

Sauce for a Cod's Head.

Take a little white Gravy, about a Pint of Oysters or Cockles, a little shred Lemon-peel, two or three Spoonfuls of White-wine, and about half a Pound of Butter thicken'd with Flour, and put it into your Boat or Bason.

To stew Oysters.

Plump them in their own Liquor, then strain them off, and wash them in cold Water; then set on a little of their own Liquor, Water, and White-wine, a Blade of Mace, and a little whole Pepper; let it boil very well, then put in your Oysters, and let them just boil up; then thicken with the Yolks of Eggs, a Piece of Butter, and a little Flour, beat up very well. Serve up with Sippets and Lemon.

Oysters in Scallop-Shells.

Take half a dozen small Scallop-Shells, lay in the Bottom of every Shell a Lump of Butter, a few Crumbs of Bread, and then your Oysters; laying over them again a few more Bread-Crumbs, a little Butter, and a little beaten Pepper; so set them to crisp, either in the Oven or before the Fire, and serve them up. They are proper either for a Side-dish or Middle-dish.

To stew Carp or Tench.

Take your Carp or Tench, and wash them; scale the Carp, but not the Tench; when you have cleaned them, wipe them with a Cloth, and fry them in a Frying-pan, with a little Butter to harden the Skin. Before you put them into the Stewpan, put to them a little good Gravy; the Quantity must be according to the Largeness of your Fish; with a Gill of Claret, three or four Anchovies at least, a little shred Lemon-peel, and a Blade or two of Mace; let all stew together till your Carp be enough, over a slow Fire; when it is enough, take Part of the Liquor, put to it half a Pound of Butter, and thicken it with a little Flour; so serve them up. Garnish your Dish with crisp Parsley, Slices of Lemon, and Pickles.

If you have not the Convenience of stewing them, you may broil them before the Fire, only adding the same Sauce.

To fry Trout, or any other Sort of Fish.

Take two or three Eggs, more or less, according as you have Fish to fry; take the Fish, and cut it in thin Slices, lay it upon a Board, rub the Eggs over it with a Feather, and strew on a little Flour and Salt; fry it in fine Dripping, or Butter; let the Dripping be very hot before you put in the Fish, but do not let it burn; if you do, it will make the Fish black. When the Fish is in the Pan, you may do the other Side with the Egg, and, as you fry it, lay it to drain before the Fire till all be fried. Then it is ready for Use.

To collar Eels.

Take the largest Eels you can get, skin and split them down the Belly, take out the Bones, season them with a little Mace, Nutmeg, and Salt; begin at the Tail, and roll them up very tight, so bind them up in a little coarse Incle, boil it in Salt and Water, with a few Bay-leaves, a little whole Pepper, and a little Alegar or Vinegar. It will take an Hour boiling, according as your Roll is in Bigness.

Bigness. When it is boiled, you must tie it, and hang it up till it be cold; then put it into the Liquor that it was boiled in, and keep it for Use.

If your Eels be small, you may roll two or three of them together.

To roast a Pike with a Pudding in the Belly.

Take a large Pike, scale and clean it; draw it at the Gills. —— To make a Pudding for the Pike. Take a large Handful of Bread-crumbs, as much Beef-Suet shred fine, two Eggs, a little Pepper and Salt, a little grated Nutmeg, a little Parsley, Sweet-marjoram, and Lemon-peel, shred fine; mix all together, put it into the Belly of your Pike, skewer it round, and lay it in an earthen Dish, with a Lump of Butter over it, a little Salt and Flour, so set it in the Oven. An Hour will roast it.

To stew a Pike.

Take a large Pike, scale and clean it, season it in the Belly with a little Mace and Salt; skewer it round, put it into a deep Stewpan, with a Pint of small Gravy, a Pint of Claret, and two or three Blades of Mace; set it over a Stove with a slow Fire, and cover it up close; when it is enough take Part of the Liquor, put to it two Anchovies, a little Lemon-peel shred fine, and thicken the Sauce with Flour and Butter. Before you lay the Pike on the Dish, turn it with the Back upwards, take off the Skin, and serve it up. Garnish your Dish with Lemon and Pickle.

Sauce for a Pike.

Take a little of the Liquor that comes from the Pike when you take it out of the Oven, put to it two or three Anchovies, a little Lemon-peel shred, a Spoonful or two of White-wine, or a little Juice of Lemon, which you please; put to it some Butter and Flour, make your Sauce about the Thickness of Cream, pour it into a Bason or Silver Boat, and set it in the Dish with your Pike. You may lay round your Pike any Sort of fried Fish, or broiled,

ed, if you have it. You may have the same Sauce for a broiled Pike, only add a little good Gravy, a few shred Capers, a little Parsley, and a Spoonful or two of Oyster or Cockle Pickle, if you have it.

To stew Eels.

Take your Eels, case, clean, and skewer them round; put them into a Stewpan, with a little good Gravy, a little Claret to redden the Gravy, a Blade or two of Mace, an Anchovy, and a little **Lemon-peel**. When they are enough, thicken with a little Flour and Butter. Garnish with Parsley.

To make Sauce for a boiled Salmon or Turbot.

Take a little mild white Gravy, two or three Anchovies, a Spoonful of Oyster or Cockle Pickle, a little shred Lemon-peel, half a Pound of Butter, a little Parsley and Fennel shred small, and a little Juice of Lemon, but not too much, for fear it should take off the Sweetness.

To make Sauce for Haddock or Cod, either broiled or boiled.

Take a little Gravy, a few Cockles, Oysters, or Mushrooms; put to them a little of the Gravy that comes from the Fish either broiled or boiled, (it will do very well if you have no other Gravy) a little Catchup, and a Lump of Butter. If you have neither Oysters nor Cockles, you may put in an Anchovy or two, and thicken it with Flour. You may put in a few shred Capers, or a little Mango, if you have it.

To make Pike eat like Sturgeon.

Take the thick Part of a large Pike, and scale it; set on two Quarts of Water to boil it in, put in a Gill of Vinegar, a large Handful of Salt, and when it boils put in your Pike, but first bind it about with coarse Incle; when it is boiled, you must not take off the Incle, but let it be on all the time it is eating. It must be kept in the same Pickle it was boiled in; and if you do not think it strong enough, you must add a little more Salt and Vinegar; so

when

when it is cold, put it upon your Pike, and keep it for Ufe. Before you boil the Pike, take out the Bone. You may do Scate the fame Way, and in my Opinion it eats more like Sturgeon.

To make Sauce for Salmon or Turbot.

Boil your Turbot or Salmon, and fet it to drain; take the Gravy that drains from the Salmon or Turbot, an Anchovy or two, a little Lemon-peel fhred, a Spoonful of Catchup, and a little Butter; thicken it with Flour the Thicknefs of Cream; put to it a little fhred Parfley and Fennel, but do not put in your Parfley and Fennel till you are juft going to fend it up, for it will take off the Green.

The Gravy of all Sorts of Fifh is a great Addition to your Sauce, if your Fifh be fweet.

To drefs Cod's Zoons.

Lay them in Water all Night, and then boil them; if they be falt, fhift them once in the boiling; when they are tender cut them in long Pieces; drefs them up with Eggs, as you do Salt-fifh; take one or two of them, and cut into fquare Pieces; dip them in Egg, and fry them to lay round the Difh.

This is proper to lay round any other Difh.

To ftew Trout.

Take a large Trout, wafh it, and put it in a Pan with White-wine and Gravy; then take two Eggs buttered, fome Pepper, Salt, Nutmeg, and Lemon-peel, a little Thyme, and fome grated Bread; mix them all together, and put in the Belly of the Trout; then let it ftew a Quarter of an Hour, and put a Piece of Butter into the Sauce; ferve it hot, and garnifh with Lemon fliced.

To ftew Cod.

Lay your Cod in thin Slices at the Bottom of your Difh, with half a Pint of White-wine, a Pint of Gravy, fome Oyfters and their Liquor, fome Pepper and Salt, and a little Nutmeg, and let it ftew till it is near enough; then

thicken

thicken it with a Piece of Butter rolled in Flour, and let it ſtew a little longer. Serve it hot, and garniſh your Diſh with Lemon ſliced.

To boil Tench.

Scale your Tench when alive, gut it, and waſh the Inſide with Vinegar; then put it into a Stewpan when the Water boils, with ſome Salt, a Bunch of Sweet-Herbs, ſome Lemon-peel, and whole Pepper; cover it up cloſe, and boil it quick till enough; then ſtrain off ſome of the Liquor, and put to it a little White-wine, ſome Walnut-Liquor, or Muſhroom Gravy, an Anchovy, and ſome Oyſters or Shrimps; boil them together, and toſs them up with thick Butter rolled in Flour, adding a little Lemon Juice. Garniſh with Lemon and Horſe-radiſh, and ſerve it up with Sippets.

To butter Shrimps.

Stew a Quart of Shrimps with half a Pint of White-wine, with a Nutmeg; then beat four Eggs with a little White-wine, and a Quarter of a Pound of beaten Butter; ſhake them well in a Diſh till they be thick enough, and ſerve them up with one Sippet for a Side-diſh.

Craw-Fiſh Soop.

Take a Knuckle of Veal, and Part of a Neck of Mutton, to make white Gravy; put in an Onion, and a little whole Pepper and Salt to your Taſte; then take twenty Craw-fiſh, boil and beat them in a Marble Mortar, adding thereto a little Gravy; ſtrain them, and put them into the Gravy, alſo two or three Pieces of white Bread to thicken the Soop. Boil twelve or fourteen of the ſmalleſt Craw-fiſh, and put them whole into the Diſh, with a few Toaſts or *French* Rolls, which you pleaſe; ſo ſerve it up.

You may make Lobſter Soop the ſame Way, only adding to it the Seeds of the Lobſter.

To collar Salmon.

Take the Side of a middling Salmon, and cut off the Head; take out all the Bones, and ſcrape the Outſide; ſeaſon

season it with Mace, Nutmeg, Pepper and Salt; roll it up tight in a Cloth, boil it, and bind it up with Incle; it will take about an Hour boiling. When it is boiled, bind it tight again; when cold, take it very carefully out of the Cloth, and bind it about with Filleting. You muſt not take off the Filleting, but as it is eaten.

To make Pickle to keep it in.

Take two or three Quarts of Water, a Gill of Vinegar, a little *Jamaica* Pepper and whole Pepper, a large Handful of Salt; boil them all together, and when it is cold put in your Salmon, ſo keep it for Uſe. If your Pickle do not keep, you muſt renew it.

You may collar Pike the ſame Way.

To roaſt a Lobſter.

If your Lobſter be alive, tie it to the Spit, roaſt and baſte it about half an Hour; if it be boiled, you muſt put it in boiling Water, and let it have a Boil, then lay it in a Dripping-pan, and baſte it. When you lay it upon the Diſh, ſplit the Tail, and lay it on each Side; ſo ſerve it up, with a little melted Butter, in a China Cup.

To butter a Crab or Lobſter.

Take all the Meat out of the Belly and Claws of your Lobſter, put it into a Stewpan, with two or three Spoonfuls of Water, a Spoonful or two of White-wine Vinegar, a little Pepper, ſhred Mace, and a Lump of Butter; ſhake it over the Stove till it be very hot, but do not let it boil; if you do, it will oil; put it into your Diſh, and lay round it your ſmall Claws. It is as proper to put it in Scallop-Shells, as on a Diſh.

To make an Oyſter Pie.

Take a Pint of the largeſt Oyſters you can get, clean them very well in their own Liquor; if you have not Liquor enough, add to them three or four Spoonfuls of Water; take the Kidney of a Loin of Veal, cut it in thin Slices, and ſeaſon it with a little Pepper and Salt; lay the

Slices

Slices in the Bottom of the Dish, (but there must be no Paste in the Bottom) cover them with the Oysters, strew over a little of the Seasoning you did for the Veal; take the Marrow of one or two Bones, lay it over your Oysters, and cover them with Puff-paste. When it is baked, take off the Lid, put into it a Spoonful or two of White-wine, shake it up all together, and serve it up. It is proper for a Side-dish, either for Noon or Night.

To broil Beef-Steaks.

Take your Steaks, and beat them with the Back of a Knife, strew them over with a little Pepper and Salt, lay them on a Gridiron over a clear Fire, turning them till they are enough; set your Dish over a Chafing-dish of Coals, with a little brown Gravy; chop an Onion small and put it amongst the Gravy; (if your Steaks be not over-much done, Gravy will come therefrom) put it on a Dish, and shake it all together. Garnish your Dish with Shalots and Pickles.

To fry Beef Steaks.

Take your Steaks and beat them with the Back of a Knife, fry them in Butter over a quick Fire, that they may be brown before they be too much done. When they are enough, put them into an earthen Pot till you have fried them all; pour out the Fat, and put them into your Pan with a little Gravy, an Onion shred very small, a Spoonful of Catchup, and a little Salt; thicken it with a little Butter and Flour the Thickness of Cream. Garnish your Dish with Pickles.

Beef Steaks are proper for a Side-dish.

To broil Beef Steaks with Oyster Sauce.

Take some tender Beef-Steaks, pepper them to your Mind, but no Salt, for that will make them hard; turn them often, till they are enough, which you will know by their feeling firm; then salt them to your Mind. For the Sauce take Oysters with their Liquor, and wash them in Salt and Water. Let the Oyster-Liquor stand to settle, and

and then pour off the Clear; stew them gently in this with a little Nutmeg or Mace, some whole Pepper, a Clove or two, and take care you do not stew them too much, for that will make them hard. When they are almost enough, add a little White-wine, and a Piece of Butter rolled in Flour to thicken it.

Some chuse to put an Anchovy, or Mushroom Catchup, into the Sauce, which makes it very rich.

To stew Beef Steaks.

Pepper and salt your Steaks, which must be cut off from the Rump, and lay them in your Stewpan; pour in about half a Pint of Water, a Blade or two of Mace, two or three Cloves, a Bunch of sweet Herbs, a Lump of Butter rolled in Flour, an Anchovy, an Onion, and a Glass of White-wine; cover them close, and let them stew softly till they are perfectly tender; then take them out of the Pan to flour them, and fry them in fresh Butter. Pour off all the Fat, strain the Sauce they were stewed in, and then pour it into the Pan; toss up all together, till you find the Sauce is both thick and hot.

To dress Veal Cutlets.

Having cut Veal in Slices, season it with Salt, Pepper, Nutmeg, Sweet Marjoram, and a little Lemon-peel grated; wash them over with Egg, and strew over them this Mixture; lard them with Bacon, dip them in melted Butter, and wrap them in white Papers butter'd; broil them on a Gridiron, a good Distance from the Fire; when they are enough, unpaper them, and serve them with Gravy, and Lemon sliced.

Another Way to dress Veal Cutlets.

Take a Neck of Veal, cut it in Joints, and flatten them with a Bill; cut off the Ends of the Bones, and lard the thick Ends of the Cutlets with four or five Bits of Bacon; season them with Nutmeg, Pepper, and Salt; strew over them a few Bread-crumbs, and sweet Herbs shred fine; first dip the Cutlets in Eggs to make the Crumbs stick, then broil

broil them before the Fire, put to them a little brown Gravy Sauce; so serve it up. Garnish your Dish with Lemon.

To fry Calves Feet in Eggs.

Boil your Calves Feet fit for eating, take out the long Bones and split them in two; when they are cold, season them with a little Pepper, Salt, and Nutmeg; take three Eggs, put to them a Spoonful of Flour, dip the Feet in it, and fry them in Butter. You must have a little Gravy and Butter for Sauce. Garnish with Currants, so serve them up.

To broil Mutton Chops.

Let your Fire be brisk and clear, then take a Loin of Mutton and cut it into Chops; pepper and salt them, and lay them on the Gridiron; keep them often turning, lest the Fat flare and black them. When you think them enough, lay them in a Dish, and send them to Table with pickled Cucumbers or Walnuts.

To fry Mutton Steaks.

Take a Loin of Mutton, cut off the thin Part, then cut the rest into Steaks, and flat them with a Bill; season them with a little Pepper and salt, fry them in Butter over a quick Fire; as you fry them put them into a Stew or Earthen Pan, till you have fried them all; then pour the Fat out of the Pan, put in a little Gravy, and the Gravy that comes from the Steaks, with a Spoonful of Claret, an Anchovy, and an Onion or a Shalot shred; shake up the Steaks in the Gravy, thicken it with a little Flour, so serve them up. Garnish with Horse-radish and Shalots.

To dress Mutton Cutlets.

Take a Handful of grated Bread, a little Thyme and Parsley and Lemon-peel shred very small, with some Nutmeg, Pepper and Salt; then take a Loin of Mutton, cut it into Steaks, and let them be well beaten; then take the Yolks of two Eggs, rub all over the Steaks, strew on the grated Bread with these Ingredients mixed; make your

Sauce

Sauce of Gravy, with a Spoonful or two of Claret, and a little Anchovy.

To broil Pigeons whole.

Take your Pigeons, ſeaſon and ſtuff them as you do jugged Pigeons, that is, take the Livers and ſhred them with Beef-ſuet, Bread-crumbs, Parſley, Sweet-marjoram, and two Eggs. Broil them either before the Fire, or in an Oven; when they are enough, take the Gravy from them, and take off the Fat; then put to the Gravy two or three Spoonfuls of Water, a little boiled Parſley ſhred, and thicken your Sauce. Garniſh your Diſh with criſp Parſley.

To broil Cod-Sounds.

After letting them lie in hot Water a few Minutes, take them out, and rub them well with Salt, to take off the black Dirt and Skin. When they look white, put them in Water, and give them a Boil; take them out and flour them well; ſalt, pepper, and broil them; when they are enough, lay them in your Diſh, and pour melted Butter and Muſtard on them. Broil them whole.

To broil Chickens.

Slit them down the Back, and ſeaſon them with Pepper and Salt; lay them over a very clear Fire, and at a great Diſtance. Let the Inſide lie next the Fire till it is above half done; then turn them, and take great Care the fleſhy Side do not burn; throw ſome fine Raſpings of Bread over it, and let them be of a fine Brown, but not burnt. Let your Sauce be good Gravy, with Muſhrooms; and garniſh with Lemon, and the Gizzards cut, ſlaſhed, and broiled with Pepper and Salt.

To broil Sauſages.

Parboil them, then take care to have a clear Fire, and your Gridiron well cleaned; that they may not ſtick, flour them well, and keep them often turning; and when you think them enough, ſerve them up to Table with Muſtard.

To broil Pork Steaks.

Let your Fire be clear and brisk, then take your Steaks, salt and pepper them well; keep them often turning, and be sure they are well done, for Pork takes more doing any other Sort of Meat.

To fry Tripe.

Cut your Tripe into Pieces about three or four Inches long, dip them in the Yolk of an Egg and a few Crumbs of Bread; fry them very brown, then take them out of your Pan, and lay them in a Dish to drain. Have another Dish warm, ready to put them in, and serve them up, with Butter and Mustard in a Cup.

To make white Scotch Collops.

Take about four Pounds of a Fillet of Veal, cut it in small Pieces as thin as you can; then take a Stewpan, butter it well over, and shake a little Flour over it, then lay your Meat in piece by piece, till all your Pan be covered; take two or three Blades of Mace and a little Nutmeg, set your Stewpan over the Fire, toss it up together till all your Meat be white; then take half a Pint of strong Veal Broth, which must be ready made, a Quarter of a Pint of Cream, and the Yolks of two Eggs; mix all these together, put it to your Meat, keeping it tossing all the Time till they just boil up; then they are enough: The last Thing you do is to squeeze in a little Lemon. You may put in Oysters, Mushrooms, or what you will, to make it rich.

To hash a Calf's-Head.

After your Calf's-Head is slit, cleansed, and half boiled and cold, cut it in thin Slices, and fry it in a Pan of brown Butter; then have a Toss-pan on the Stove, with a Pint of Gravy, as much strong Broth, a Quarter of a Pint of Claret, as much White-wine, and a Handful of savoury Balls, two or three shrivelled Palates, a Pint of Oysters, Cock's-combs, Lamb-stones, and Sweet-breads, boiled, blanched,

blanched, and sliced, with Mushrooms and Truffles; then put your Hash in the Dish, and the other Things, some round, and some on it. Garnish your Dish with Lemon.

To hash Beef.

Cut some Slices of tender Beef, and put them into a Stewpan well floured, with a Slice of Butter, over a quick Fire, for three Minutes; and then put to them a little Water, a Bunch of sweet Herbs, or a little Marjoram alone, an Onion, some Lemon-peel, with some Pepper, Salt, and some Nutmeg grated. Cover these close, and let them stew till they are tender; then put in a Glass of Claret, or Beer that is not bitter, and strain your Sauce; serve it up hot, and garnish it with red Beet Roots and Lemon sliced. This is a very good Dish.

A fine Hash of Beef, at little Expence.

After having cut your Beef in thin Slices, make your Sauce for it as follows: Take some Pepper and Salt, an Onion cut in two, a little Water, and some strong Beer; after that take a Piece of Butter rolled in Flour, put it in your Pan, stirring it till it burns; then put in your Sauce, and let it boil a Minute or two; then put in your Beef, and let it but just warm through, for it will harden it if you let it lie too long. You may put in a little Claret just before you take it off the Fire; if you use no Beer, take some Mushroom or Walnut Liquor. Garnish with Pickles.

To hash a Leg of Mutton.

Take a Leg of Mutton half roasted; when it is cold, cut it in thin Pieces, as you would do any other Meat for hashing; put it into a Stewpan, with a little Water or small Gravy, two or three Spoonfuls of Red Wine, two or three Shalots shred, or Onions, and some Oyster-Pickle; thicken it with a little Flour, and so serve it up. Garnish your Dish with Horse-radish and Pickles. You may do a Shoulder of Mutton the same Way, only boil the Bladebone, and let it lie in the Middle of the Dish.

To hash Mutton.

Cut your Mutton in small Pieces, and then take about half a Pint of Oysters, and, after washing them in Water, put them in their own Liquor in a Saucepan, with some Mace, whole Pepper, and a little Salt. When they have stewed a little, put in one Anchovy, a Spoonful of Kitchen Sauce or pickled Walnut Liquor, some Gravy, or Water; then put in your Mutton, and a piece of Butter rolled in Flour; let it boil up till the Mutton is warm through, then put in Glass of Claret; lay it upon Sippets, garnish with sliced Lemon or Capers, and, if you please, some Mushrooms.

Another Way to hash Mutton, or any such Meat.

Take a little Pepper, whole Mace, Salt, a few Sprigs of sweet Herbs, a little Anchovy, one Shalot, two Slices of Lemon, and a little Broth or Water; let it stew a little, thicken it with burnt Butter, and serve it up with Pickles and Sippets.

To stew a Fillet of Veal.

Take a Leg of the best white Veal, cut off the Dug and the Knuckle, cut the rest into two Fillets; take the fat Part, and cut it in Pieces the Thickness of your Finger; you must stuff the Veal with the Fat; make a Hole with a Penknife, draw it through, and skewer it round; season it with Pepper, Salt, Nutmeg, and shred Parsley; then put it into your Stewpan, with half a Pound of Butter, (without Water) and set it on your Stove; let it boil very slow, and cover it close up, turning it very often; it will take about two Hours in stewing. When it is enough pour the Gravy from it, take off the Fat, put into the Gravy a Pint of Oysters, and a few Capers, a little Lemon-peel, a Spoonful or two of White-wine, and a little Juice of Lemon; thicken it with Butter and Flour the Thickness of Cream; lay round it Forced-meat Balls and Oysters fried; serve it up, and garnish your Dish with a few Capers and sliced Lemon.

To stew a Rump of Beef.

Take a fat Rump of young Beef, and cut off the fag End; lard the low Part with fat Bacon, and stuff the other Part with shred Parsley; put it into your Pan with two or three Quarts of Water, a Quart of Red Wine, two or three Anchovies, an Onion, two or three Blades of Mace, a little whole Pepper, and a Bunch of sweet Herbs; stew it over a slow Fire five or six Hours, turning it several Times in the stewing, and keep it close covered. When your Beef is stewed enough, take from it the Gravy, thicken part of it with a Lump of Butter and Flour, and put it upon the Dish with the Beef. Garnish the Dish with Horse-radish and red Beet-root. There must be no Salt upon the Beef, only salt the Gravy to your Taste.

You may stew part of a Brisket or an Ox-Cheek the same Way.

To stew Beef Collops.

Cut raw Beef in the same Manner as you do Veal for *Scotch* Collops; lay it in a Dish with a little Water, put to it a Shalot, a Glass of White-wine, some Marjoram powdered, some Pepper and Salt, and a Slice of fat Bacon; then put it over a quick Fire for a little Time, till your Dish is full of Gravy, and you may put in a little Catchup. Serve it hot, and garnish with Lemon-peel sliced.

To stew Pigeons.

Take your Pigeons, season and stuff them, flat the Breast-bone, and truss them up as you would do for baking; dredge them over with a little Flour, and fry them in Butter, turning them round till all Sides be brown; then put them into a Stewpan with as much brown Gravy as will cover them, and let them stew till they are enough; then take part of the Gravy, an Anchovy shred, a little Catchup, a small Onion or a Shalot, and a little Juice of Lemon for Sauce; pour it over your Pigeons, and lay round them

Forced-

Forced-meat Balls and crisp Bacon. Garnish your Dish with crisp Parsley and Lemon.

To stew Ducks whole.

Take Ducks when they are drawn and clean washed, put them into a Stewpan with strong Broth, Red Wine, Mace, whole Pepper, an Onion, an Anchovy, and Lemon-peel; when well stewed, put in a Piece of Butter and some grated Bread to thicken it; lay round them crisp Bacon, and Forced-meat Balls. Garnish with Shalots.

To stew a Hare.

Take a young Hare, wash and wipe it well, cut the Legs into two or three Pieces, and all the other Parts of the same Bigness; beat them all flat with a Paste-pin, season it with Nutmeg and Salt, then flour it over, and fry it in Butter over a quick Fire. When you have fried it, put it into a Stewpan, with a Pint of Gravy, two or three Spoonfuls of Claret, and a small Anchovy; so shake it up with Butter and Flour, (you must not let it boil in the Stewpan, for it will make it eat hard) then serve it up. Garnish your Dish with crisp Parsley.

To stew Ducks wild or tame.

Take two Ducks and half roast them, cut them up as you would do for eating, put them into a Stewpan with a little brown Gravy, a Glass of Claret, two Anchovies, a small Onion shred very fine, and a little Salt; thicken it with Flour and Butter, so serve it up. Garnish your Dish with Onion Sippets.

To stew a Rump, Leg, or Neck of Mutton.

First break the Bones, and put them in a Pot, with a little whole Pepper, Mace and Salt, one Anchovy, one Nutmeg, and one Turnip, two Onions, a little Bunch of sweet Herbs, a Pint of Ale, a Quart of Claret, a Quart or two of Water, and a hard Crust of Bread; stop it up, and let it stew five Hours, and serve it up with Toasts and the Gravy. Put half this to the Mutton, and stew it two Hours. You may bake an Ox-Cheek in the same Manner.

To stew Mutton Chops.

Cut your Chops thin, take two earthen Pans, put one over the other, lay your Chops between them, and burn brown Paper under them.

To stew Rabbets.

Take two or three Rabbets, and after boiling them till they are half done, cut them into Pieces in the Joints, and cut the Meat off in Pieces, leaving some Meat on the Bones; then put Bones and Meat in o a good Quantity of the Liquor in which the Rabbets were parboiled; set it over a Chafing-dish of Coals between two Dishes, and let it stew; season it with Salt and grofs Pepper, and then put in some Oil; and before you take it off the Fire, squeeze in some Juice of Lemon. When it has stewed enough, serve it up all together in the Dish.

To stew Rabbets the French Way.

Cut your Rabbets into Quarters, then lard them with pretty large Lardoons of Bacon, fry them, stew them in a Stewpan with strong Broth, White-wine, Pepper, Salt, a Faggot of sweet Herbs, fried Flour, and Orange.

To stew a Pig.

In the first place, roast the Pig till it is hot; then take off the Skin, and cut it in pieces; then put it into a Stewpan, with good Gravy and White-wine, some Pepper, Salt, Nutmeg, and Onion, a little sweet Marjoram, a little Elder Vinegar, and some Butter; and when it is enough, lay it upon Sippets, and garnish with sliced Lemon.

To stew Eggs in Gravy.

Take a little Gravy, pour it upon a little Pewter Dish, and set it over a Stove; when it is hot, break in as many Eggs as will cover the Bottom of the Dish; keep pouring the Gravy over them with a Spoon till they are white at the Top, and when they are done enough, ſtrew over them a little Salt; fry ſome ſquare Sippets of Bread in Butter, prick them with the ſmall End upwards, and ſerve them up.

To bake a Pig.

Lay it in a Diſh, and flour it well; then rub it all over with Butter: The Diſh you lay it in muſt alſo be well butter'd. Thus prepared ſend it to the Oven; as ſoon as it is drawn, if enough, rub it over with a Cloth well butter'd; then ſet it in the Oven again till it is dry. Take it out, and put it in a Diſh; then cut it up; take a little Gravy made of Veal, and take off the Fat that lay in the Diſh it was baked in, and you will find a ſmall Quantity of good Gravy at the Bottom; put that to your Veal Gravy, with the Addition of a Lump of Butter rolled in Flour; when you have boiled your Gravy up, put it into your Diſh, and intermingle it with the Brains and the Sage that were baked in the Belly of it. If you chuſe to have the Pig ſerved up to the Table whole, you have nothing more to do than put ſuch Sauce into the Diſh as you judge moſt proper.

To bake a Calf's-Head.

Pick it, and waſh it very clean; let your Diſh be large enough for the Purpoſe; rub ſome Butter all over the Diſh, then lay ſeveral Iron Skewers acroſs the Top of it, and your Head upon them; ſkewer up your Meat in the Middle, ſo that it may not lie in the Diſh; then grate ſome Nutmeg all over it, add to this ſome ſweet Herbs ſhred very ſmall, ſome Crumbs of Bread, a little Lemon-peel ſhred ſmall, and then duſt it over with Flour; ſtick little Lumps of Butter into the Eyes, and all over the Head, and then flour it once more: Take care that it be well baked, and of a fine Brown. If you pleaſe, you may ſtrew a ſmall Quantity of Pepper and Salt over it, and put a Piece of Beef ſhred ſmall into your Diſh, a Bunch of ſweet Herbs, one Onion, ſome whole Pepper, a Blade of Mace, two Cloves, about a Pint of Water, and boil your Brains with a small Quantity of Sage. When it is baked enough, lay it in a Dish, and set it before the Fire; then stir all together in the Dish, and boil it in a Saucepan; strain it off, then put it into the Saucepan once more, add thereto a Lump of Butter rolled in Flour, and the Sage in the Brains chopp'd fine, two Spoonfuls of Red Wine, and one of Catchup; boil them all together, then beat the Brains well, and mingle them with the Sauce; pour it all into the Dish; and serve it up. Take notice, you must bake the Tongue with the Head, and not cut it out. Bake a Sheep's-Head the same Way.

To bake Mutton Chops.

Strew some Pepper and Salt over them; butter your Dish, and lay in your Steaks: Then take a Quart of Milk, beat up six Eggs very fine, and add to this four Spoonfuls of Flour; beat your Flour and Eggs first in a little Milk, and put the rest to it; put in likewise a little beaten Ginger; pour this all over your Chops, and send it to the Oven, where you must let it stand about an Hour and a half.

To bake Ox-Palates.

After you have salted a Tongue, cut off the Root, and take some Ox-Palates, and wash them clean; then cut them into several Pieces, put them into an earthen Pan, cover them over with Water, and put in a Blade or two of Mace, about a Dozen whole Pepper-Corns, three Cloves, a small Bunch of sweet Herbs, a small Onion, and half a Spoonful of Raspings; cover it close with brown Paper, and let it be well baked. When it comes from the Oven, season it as you like it.

To bake a Leg of Beef.

When it is baked, pick out all the Sinews and Fat, put them into a Saucepan with a few Spoonfuls of the Gravy, a Glass of Red Wine, and a Lump of Butter rolled in Flour; add to it a little Mustard; shake your Saucepan often,

often, and when it is hot, and pretty thick, serve it up to Table.

To bake Beef the French Way.

Bone some tender Beef, take away the Sinews and Skin, then lard it with fat Bacon; season your Beef with Salt, Pepper and Cloves, then tie it up tight with Packthread, and put it into an earthen Pan, with some whole Pepper, and an Onion stuck with twelve Cloves; and put at Top a Bunch of sweet Herbs, two or three Bay-leaves, a Quarter of a Pound of Butter, and half a Pint of Claret, or White-wine Vinegar or Verjuice; cover it close, and bake it for four or five Hours; serve it hot with its own Liquor, or cold in Slices, to be eat with Vinegar and Mustard.

To bake Lamb with Rice.

Half roast your Loin or Neck of Lamb, then take it up, and cut it into Steaks; after that, take about half a Pound of Rice, put it into about a Quart of good Gravy, with a few Blades of Mace and a little Nutmeg; do it over a slow Fire or Stove till your Rice begins to be thick; when you have taken it off, stir a Pound of Butter into it, and when perfectly melted stir in the Yolks of half a Dozen Eggs, but beat them first; then butter your Dish all over, pepper and salt your Steaks, dip them in a little melted Butter, lay them into the Dish, pour the Gravy which comes off them all over them, and after that the Rice; beat the Yolks of three Eggs, and pour all over; send it thus prepared to the Oven, and it will be enough if you let it stay in something better than half an Hour.

To bake Herrings and Sprats.

Put a hundred Herrings into a Pan, cover them with three Parts Water and one Part Vinegar, with a good deal of All Spice, some Cloves, a Bunch of sweet Herbs, a few Bay-leaves, and two whole Onions; tie them down close and bake them; when they come out of the Oven, heat a Pint of Red Wine scalding hot, and put to them; then

then tie them down again, and let them stand four or five Days before you open them, and they will be very firm and fine.

FRICASSEES.

How to fricaſſee Rabbets brown.

TAKE a Rabbet, cut the Legs into three Pieces, and the Remainder of the Rabbet the same Bigneſs, beat them thin, and fry them in Butter over a quick Fire; when they are fried put them into a Stewpan with a little Gravy, a Spoonful of Catchup, and a little Nutmeg; then ſhake it up with a little Flour and Butter. Garniſh your Diſh with criſp Parſley.

To make a white Fricaſſee of Rabbets

Take a Couple of young Rabbets, and half roaſt them; when they are cold take off the Skin, and cut the Rabbets in ſmall Pieces, (only take the white Part) put them into a Stewpan with white Gravy, a ſmall Anchovy, a little Onion, ſhred Mace and Lemon-peel; ſet it over a Stove, and let it have one Boil; then take a little Cream, the Yolks of two Eggs, a Lump of Butter, a little Juice of Lemon and ſhred Parſley; put them all together into a Stewpan, and ſhake them over the Fire till they be as white as Cream; you muſt not let it boil, if you do it will curdle. Garniſh your Diſh with ſhred Lemon and Pickles.

To make a white Fricaſſee of Chickens.

Take two or more Chickens, half roaſt them, cut them up as you would do for eating, and ſkin them; put them into a Stewpan with a little white Gravy, Juice of Lemon, two Anchovies, ſhred Mace, and Nutmeg, and boil it; take the Yolks of three Eggs, a little ſweet Cream and ſhred Parſley; put them into your Stewpan with a Lump of Butter and a little Salt, ſhake them all the while they over the Stove, and be sure you do not let them boil, lest they should curdle. Garnish your Dish with Sippets and Lemon.

To make a brown Fricassee of Chickens.

Take two or more Chickens, as you would have your Dish in Bigness, cut them up as you do for eating, and flat them a little with a Paste-pin; fry them a light Brown, and put them into your Stewpan with a little Gravy, a Spoonful or two of White-wine, a little Nutmeg and Salt; thicken it up with Flour and Butter. Garnish your Dish with Sippets and crisp Parsley.

To make a Fricassee of Tripe.

Take the whitest seam Tripe you can get, and cut it in long Pieces; put them into a Stewpan, with a little good Gravy, a few Bread-crumbs, a Lump of Butter, a little Vinegar to your Taste, and a little Mustard if you like it; shake it up all together with a little shred Parsley. Garnish your Dish with Sippets.

This is proper for a Side-dish.

To make a Fricassee of Veal Sweetbreads.

Take five or six Veal Sweetbreads, according as you would have your Dish in Bigness, and boil them in Water; cut them in thin Slices the length Way, dip them in Eggs, season them with Pepper and Salt; fry them a light Brown; then put them into a Stewpan, with a little brown Gravy, a Spoonful of White-wine or Juice of Lemon, which you please; thicken it up with Flour and Butter, and serve it up. Garnish your Dish with crisp Parsley

To fricassee Lamb.

Take a hind Quarter of Lamb, and cut it into thin Slices; season them with savoury Spice, sweet Herbs, and a Shalot; then fry them on the Fire, toss them up in strong Broth, Oysters, White-wine Forced-meat Balls, two Palates, a little brown Butter, and an Egg or two to thicken

it,

The Young Woman's best Companion. 53

it, or a bit of Butter rolled in Flour. Garnish your Dish with sliced Lemon.

To make a white Fricassee of Tripe to eat like Chickens.

Take the whitest and the thickest seam Tripe you can get, cut the white Part in thin Slices, put it into a Stew-pan, with a little white Gravy, Juice of Lemon, and Lemon peel shred, also a Spoonful of White-wine; take the Yolks of two or three Eggs, and beat them very well, put to them a little thick Cream, shred Parsley, and two or three Chives, if you have any; shake all together over a Stove till it be as thick as Cream, but do not let it boil, for fear it curdle. Garnish your Dish with Sippets, sliced Lemon, or Mushrooms, and serve it up.

General Rules *to be observed in the making of* Soups *or* Broths.

IN the first place, be particularly careful that all your Pots, Saucepans and Covers, be perfectly clean, and free from either Grease or Sand: Take great Care likewise that they be well tinn'd, for otherwise they will give your Broths or Soups a disagreeable brassy Taste. If you are not too much hurried, stew your Meat as softly as you can; for by that means it will not only be more tender, but have a finer Flavour.

When you make Soup or Broth for immediate Use, you must stew your Meat softly, and put in but very little more Water than you intend to have Soup or Broth. If you have an earthen Pan or Pipkin, set it on Wood Embers till it boils; then skim it, and put your Seasoning into it; after that cover it close, and set it on the Embers again, that it may stew gently for some Time. This Method observed will make both your Broth and your Meat also very delicious. In all your Soups and Broths you must take care that no one of your Ingredients be predo-

F 3 minant

minant over the rest; the Taste should be equal, and the Relish agreeable to what you particularly intend it for. Take notice, that whatever Greens or Herbs you put into your Broths or Soups, they must all be well clean'd, wash'd and pick'd, before they are made use of.

To make Mutton Broth.

Take about six Pounds of a Neck of Mutton, and cut it into two Parts; boil the Crag in a Gallon of Water, and as the Scum arises take it off; then put in what Quantity of sweet Herbs you think proper, as also one Onion, and a large Crust of Bread. When your Crag has boiled for an Hour, put in the Remainder of your Meat, two or three Turnips, some Chives, and some Parsley chopp'd small; season it with Salt to your Palate. You may thicken it either with Bread and Oatmeal, Barley, or Rice, as your Inclination directs you. If you propose to have Turnips for Sauce to your Meat, do not boil the whole in your Broth, because it will make it too strong.

To make Chicken or White Broth.

Parboil a Chicken or Pullet, and when you have taken the Flesh from the Bones, put it into a Stewpan over a Chafing-dish of Coals; add to this as much boiled Cream as you shall think proper; thicken this with Flour, Rice, and Eggs, and a small Quantity of Marrow, in some of the Broth your Fowl was boiled in; then pour in about a Gill either of Sack or Mountain, and season with Salt and Pepper to your Palate. When it is thickened to your Satisfaction, serve it up to Table.

Chickens Surprise.

Take half a Pound of Rice, set it over a Fire in soft Water, when it is half boiled put in two or three small Chickens trussed, with two or three Blades of Mace, and a little Salt; take a Piece of Bacon about three Inches square, and boil it in Water till it is almost enough; take it out, pare off the Outside, and put it in to the Chickens and

and Rice to boil a little together; (you muſt not let the Broth be over thick with Rice) then take up your Chickens, lay them on a Diſh, pour over them the Rice, cut your Bacon in thin Slices to lay round your Chickens, and upon the Breaſt of each a Slice. This is proper for a Side-diſh.

To make Barley Broth.

Set three Quarts of Water upon the Fire, and put into your Saucepan a Pound of *French* Barley; when it has boiled for ſome Time, throw in ſome whole Spice, and what Quantity of Raiſins and Currants you think proper. When it is boiled enough, put a Lump of Butter and a little Roſe-Water into it; then ſweeten it to your Palate, and eat it.

To make Veal Broth.

Take a Neck of Veal, cut the Crag off, and boil it over a ſlow Fire; put into your Pan ſome Salt and Pepper, with Thyme and Parſley, and after it has boiled ſome Time, put in the Remainder of your Meat, and take care that it is boiled well; then ſerve it up to Table with melted Butter and Parſley.

To make Calves-Feet Broth.

After boiling the Feet in juſt ſo much Water as will make a good Jelly, ſtrain it, and ſet the Liquor on the Fire again, putting in two or three Blades of Mace: Put about half a Pint of Sack to two Quarts of Broth; add half a Pound of Currants picked and waſhed, and when they are plumped, beat up the Yolks of two Eggs, mix them with a little of the cold Liquor, and thicken it carefully over a gentle Fire; then ſweeten it with Sugar to your Palate, and ſeaſon it with Salt; then ſtir in a bit of Butter, with the Juice and Peel of a freſh Lemon, before you take it off.

Jelly Broth for Conſumptive Perſons.

Get a Joint of Mutton, a Capon, a Fillet of Veal, and three Quarts of Water; put theſe in an earthen Pot, and boil

boil them over a gentle Fire till one Half be confumed; then fqueeze all together, and ftrain the Liquor through a Linen Cloth.

To make a good Gravy Soup.

Boil a Leg of Beef down, with a fmall Quantity of Salt, a Bunch of fweet Herbs, a few Cloves, a bit of Nutmeg, and an Onion. Boil three Gallons of Water down to one; then cut three or four Pounds of lean Beef into thin Slices, and before you put your Meat into your Pan put in a Lump of Butter about the Bignefs of an Egg, that has been floured. When your Stewpan is hot, and your Butter is properly brown'd, lay your Meat in, and having covered it, let it ftew over a quick Fire, but take care to give it a Turn now and then; and ftrain in your ftrong Broth, with an Anchovy or two, a Handful of Endive and Spinage boiled green, drained, and fhred grofs; then have fome Palates ready boiled, cut into fmall Pieces, toafted and fried. Take out your Beef, put the Remainder all together with fome Pepper, boil it up, and ferve it with a Knuckle of Veal or a boil'd Fowl in the Middle of it.

To make green Peafe Soup.

Put a Peck of thefe Peafe into a Stewpan, and cover them with Water; then put to them fome Salt and Pepper, a few young Onions, a little Parfley, and a Bunch of Thyme; add to thefe a Quarter of a Pound of Bacon, and a good Lump of Butter; then cover them, and when they have ftewed for a fhort Time, take half a Dozen Cabbage-Lettuces, or more in cafe they are but fmall, and put them into the Soup when cut into Quarters; add to them ten or a dozen Cucumbers, or lefs in cafe they are large, with a Handful of Purflane, together with fome more Seafoning, and a large Lump of Butter: Fill your Stew-pan with boiling Water, and let your Soup ftew for two or three Hours or more; and if in that Time you find your Liquor wafted away too much, throw into it a Lump of of Butter, and as much more boiling Water as you see convenient. You may stew in this Soup, if you please, either two or three Pigeons or a Chicken, with proper Stuffing in their Bellies.

To make dried Peafe Soup.

This may be made of Beef, but a Leg of Pork is the better of the two. Strain your Broth through a Sieve, and put half a Pint of split Peafe to every Quart of Liquor, or a Quart of whole Peafe to three Quarts of Liquor. When you make use of the latter, they must be passed through a Cullender; but the former need not. Cut as much Celery into it, in little Pieces, as you think proper, a small Quantity of Marjoram in Powder, and some dried Mint. When you have seasoned it with Pepper and Salt, let it boil till your Celery is tender. Take notice, If you boil a whole Leg of Pork, this is not to be done till after your Meat is taken out of the Pot; but if you boil the Bones of Pork only, or the Hock, boil these Ingredients afterwards in the Liquor. When you serve this Soup up to Table, lay a *French* Roll in the Middle of it, and make use of rasped Bread, sifted, to garnish the Border of your Dish.

To make Peafe Pottage

Boil four Quarts of Peafe in as little Water as will be sufficient, till they are soft and duly thickened. While these are preparing, boil a Leg of Mutton and two or three Humbles of Veal in another Pot, pricking them with a Knife in order to let out the Gravy; boil them in no more Water than what will just cover them. When you have boiled out all the Goodness of your Meat, strain the Liquor, put into it the Pulp of the Peafe, and let them boil together; then put in a good Piece of Bacon, a large Bunch of Mint, and a little Thyme. As soon as it is enough, put it into your Dish, and lay small Rashers of Bacon all round it; but before you serve it up, pour a sufficient Quantity of melted Butter into it.

To make Rice Soup.

Pick and wash a Quarter of a Pound of Rice as clean as possible, and boil it in some Veal Broth till it is perfectly tender, with a Chicken, and a small Quantity of Mace; then skim it well, and season it with Salt to your Palate; then stir in half a Pound of Butter, and a Pint of Cream boiled up into your Soup. When all Things are thus prepared, serve up the Fowl and the Soup with the Crumb of a *French* Roll.

To make Onion Soup.

Put half a Pound of good Butter into a Stewpan, and let it all melt over the Fire, and boil, till it makes no manner of Noise; then take about a dozen of Onions peel'd, or less, according as they are in Bigness, and cut them small: When thus shred, throw them into your melted Butter, and let them fry for about fifteen or twenty Minutes; then, when you have shaken in a small Quantity of Flour, stir them round about, shake your Pan, and let them fry for a few Minutes longer; then add to them a Quart or more, if you think proper, of boiling Water, and stir them round once more; then throw into them a large Piece of the upper Crust of a stale Loaf, and season with Salt to your Taste: Keep them boiling for ten Minutes longer over the Fire, but let them be frequently stirred; then take them off, and have the Yolks of two Eggs beat fine with half a Spoonful of Vinegar ready to put to them; and having mingled some of your Soup with them, stir it well, and mix it well with the Remainder of your Soup, and so serve it up to Table.

To roll a Breast of Veal.

Take a Breast of Veal and bone it, season it with Nutmeg, Pepper, and Salt, rub it over with the Yolk of an Egg; then strew it over with sweet Herbs shred small, and some Slices of Bacon, cut thin, to lie upon it; roll it up very tight, bind it with coarse Incle, put it into an earthen Dish with a little Water, and lay upon it some

Lumps

Lumps of Butter; strew a little Seasoning on the Outside of your Veal: It will take two Hours baking; when it is baked take off the Incle, and cut it in four Rolls; lay it upon the Dish with a good brown Gravy Sauce, and lay about your Veal the Sweetbread fried, some Forced-meat Balls, a little crisp Bacon, and a few fried Oysters, if you have any; so serve it up. Garnish your Dish with Pickles and Lemon.

To roll a Pig's-Head to eat like Brawn.

Take a large Pig's Head, cut off the Groin Ends, crack the Bone, put it in Water, shift it once or twice, cut off the Ears, and boil it so tender that the Bones will slip out; nick it with a Knife in the thick Part of the Head, throw over it a pretty large Handful of Salt; take half a dozen large Neat's Feet, boil them till they be soft, split them, and take out all the Bones and black Bits; take a strong coarse Cloth, and lay your Feet with the Skin-side downwards, with all the loose Pieces on the Inside; press them with your Hands to make them of equal Thickness; lay them at that Length that they will reach round the Head, and throw over them a Handful of Salt; then lay your Head across, one thick Part one Way, and the other another, that the Fat may appear alike at both Ends; leave one Foot out to lay at the Top, to make the Lanthorn to reach round; bind it with Filleting as you would do Brawn, and tie it very close at both Ends. You may take it out of the Cloth the next Day; take off the Filleting and wash it, wrap it about it again very tight, and keep it in Brawn-Pickle.

This has been often taken for real Brawn.

To collar a Pig.

Take a large Pig that is fat, about a Month old, kill and dress it, cut off the Head, cut it in two down the Back, and bone it; then cut it in three or four Pieces, wash it in a little Water to take out the Blood; take a little Milk and Water just warm, put in your Pig, let it lie about

about a Day and a Night, shift it two or three Times in that Time to make it white, then take it out, and wipe it very well with a dry Cloth, and season it with Mace, Nutmeg, Pepper, and Salt; take a little shred Parsley, and sprinkle over two of the Quarters; so roll them up in a fine soft Cloth, tie it up at both Ends, bind it up tight with a little Filleting or coarse Incle, and boil it in Milk and Water with a little Salt; it will take about an Hour and a half boiling: When it is enough, bind it up tight in your Cloth again, and hang it up till it be cold. For the Pickle, boil a little Milk and Water, a few Bay-leaves, and a little Salt. When it is cold, take your Pig out of the Cloths, and put it into the Pickle; you must shift it out of your Pickle two or three Times to make it white. The last Pickle make strong, and put in a little whole Pepper, a pretty large Handful of Salt, a few Bay-leaves, and so keep it for Use.

To make Rolls of Beef.

Cut your Beef thin, as for *Scotch* Collops; beat it very well, and season it with Salt, *Jamaica* and white Pepper, Mace, Nutmeg, Sweet Marjoram, Parsley, Thyme, and a little Onion shred small; rub them on the Collops on one Side, then take long Bits of Beef-Suet, and roll in them, tying them up with a Thread; flour them well, and fry them in Butter very brown; have ready some good Gravy, and stew them an Hour and a half, stirring them often, and keep them covered. When they are enough, take off the Threads, put in a little Flour, with a good Lump of Butter, and squeeze in some Lemon; then they are ready for Use.

To collar Beef.

Strip the Skin off a thin Piece of the Flank, and then beat your Meat well with a Rolling-pin; have in Readiness a Quart of Petre-Salt that has been dissolved in five Quarts of Water and strained, and throw your Meat into it: There let it lie for five or six Days; but take care to turn

turn it every now and then. When it is thus far prepared, take a Quarter of an Ounce of Cloves, a small Quantity of Mace, with a little Pepper, and a whole Nutmeg, all beaten well together: Add to this a Handful of Thyme that has been stript off the Stalks. When you have taken your Meat out of the Brine, strew your Seasoning all over it; over that lay on the Skin that you had stript off, and roll up your Meat in it as close as possible; then tie it hard with coarse Tape, and put it into a deep Pot; and when you have added to it a Pint of Claret, send it to the Oven, and let it be well baked.

To make Dutch Beef.

Take the lean Part of a Buttock of Beef raw, rub it well with brown Sugar all over, and let it lie in a Pan or Tray two or three Hours, turning it three or four times; then salt it with common Salt, and two Ounces of Salt-petre; let it lie a Fortnight, turning it every Day; then roll it very strait, and put it into a Cheese-press a Day and a Night; then take off the Cloth, and hang it up to dry in the Chimney. When you boil it, let it be boiled very well; it will cut in Shivers like *Dutch* Beef.

You may do a Leg of Mutton the same Way.

To pot Beef.

When you have cut your Beef small, let it afterwards be well beaten in a Marble Mortar, with some Butter melted for that Purpose, and two or three Anchovies, till you find your Meat mellow and agreeable to your Palate. Thus prepared, put it close down in Pots, and pour over them a sufficient Quantity of clarified Butter. You may season your Ingredients with what Spice you please. The Inside of a Rump of Beef is generally thought to be the best for the Purpose.

To pot either Fowls or Pigeons.

When you have cut their Legs off, draw them, and wipe them well with a Cloth, but never wash them; season them with Pepper and Salt pretty high; then put them down close in a Pot, with as much Butter as you think will cover them when melted, and bake them very tender; then drain them perfectly dry from their Gravy, which is best done by laying them on a Cloth; then season them again, not only with Salt and Pepper, but with such a Quantity of Mace and Cloves, beaten very fine, as you see convenient, and then pot them again as close as you can. Clear the Butter from your Gravy when it is cold, and when you have melted it pour it over your Fowls. If you have not a sufficient Quantity, you must clarify more; for your Butter must be at least an Inch thick over your Birds. Most People bone their Wild Fowl, but that Particular is entirely left to your own Opinion.

To pot Pigeons.

Take your Pigeons, and skewer them with their Feet cross over the Breast, to stand up; season them with Pepper and Salt, and roast them; put them into your Pot, setting the Feet up; when they are cold, cover them up with clarified Butter.

To pot Smelts.

Take the freshest and largest Smelts you can get, wipe them very well with a clean Cloth, take out the Guts with a Skewer, (but you must not take out the Milt and Roe) season them with a little Mace, Nutmeg, and Salt, so lay them in a flat Pot; if you have two Score, you may lay over them five Ounces of Butter; tie over them a Paper, and set them in a slow Oven; if it be too hot, it will burn them, and make them look black; an Hour will bake them. When they are baked you must take them out, and lay them on a Dish to drain, and when they are drained you must put them in long Pots, about the Length of your Smelts. When you lay them in, you must put betwixt every Layer the Seasoning as you did before, to make them keep. When they are cold, cover them over with clarified Butter; so keep them for Use.

To pot Mushrooms.

Take the largest Mushrooms, scrape and clean them; put them into your Pan, with a Lump of Butter, and a little Salt; let them stew over a slow Fire till they are enough; put to them a little Mace and whole Pepper, then dry them with a Cloth, and put them into a Pan as close as you can, and, as you lay them down, sprinkle in a little Salt and Mace; when they are cold, cover them over with Butter. When you use them, toss them up with Gravy, a few Bread-crumbs, and Butter. Do not make your Pot too large, but rather put them in two Pots. They will keep the better, if you take the Gravy from them when they are stewed.

They are good for Fish-Sauce, or any other, while they are fresh.

To make Black Puddings.

Take two Quarts of whole Oatmeal, pick it, and half boil it; give it Room in your Cloth, (you must do it the Day before you use it) put it into the Blood till it is warm, with a Handful of Salt, stir it very well, beat eight or nine Eggs in about a Pint of Cream, and a Quart of Bread-crumbs, a Handful or two of Maslin Meal dressed through a Hair Sieve, if you have it, if not, put in Wheat Flour; to this Quantity you may put an Ounce of *Jamaica* Pepper, an Ounce of Black Pepper, a large Nutmeg, and a little more Salt, Sweet Marjoram and Thyme, if they be green, shred them fine; if dry, rub them to Powder; mix them well together, and if it be too thick, put a little Milk into it. Take four Pounds of Beef-suet, and four Pounds of Lard, skin and cut it in thin Pieces, put it into your Blood by Handfuls, as you fill your Puddings; when they are filled and tied, prick them with a Pin, it will keep them from bursting in the boiling; (you must boil them twice) cover them close, and it will make them black.

To make Black Puddings the common Way.

First, get a Peck of Groats, and boil them for an Hour and a half in Water; then drain them, and throw them into a clean earthen Pan, or clean Tub; then kill your Hog, and take two Quarts of his Blood, which must be kept constantly stirring till it is cold; then mingle it with your Groats so boiled as above mentioned, and stir all your Ingredients well together. As to your Seasoning, take one large Spoonful of Salt, a Quarter of an Ounce of Cloves, and as much Mace and Nutmeg; dry it, beat it, and mix it all well together; add to it a small Quantity of Winter-savoury, sweet Marjoram, Thyme, and Penny-royal, chopp'd as fine as possible, just to give it a Flavour. The next Day, cut the Leaf of the Hog into Squares like Dice; then wash and scrape the Guts as clean as possible, and when you have tied up one End, begin to fill them, till they are near three Parts full; but take care to mingle the Fat in due Proportion with your other Ingredients. You may make your Puddings of what Length you think proper. When they are tied, prick them with a Fork or a Pin, and throw them into a Kettle of hot Water; there let them boil gently for about an Hour, in which Time they will be enough. Then take them out, and let them dry upon clean Straw.

To make White Puddings in Skins.

Take half a Pound of Rice, cree it in Milk till it be soft; when it is creed, put it into a Cullender to drain; take a Penny-Loaf, cut off the out Crust, then cut it into thin Slices, scald it in a little Milk, but do not make it too wet; take six Eggs, and beat them very well, a Pound of Currants well cleaned, a Pound of Beef-suet shred fine, two or three Spoonfuls of Rose-water, Half a Pound of Powder Sugar, a little Salt, a Quarter of an Ounce of Mace, a large Nutmeg grated, and a small Stick of Cinnamon; beat them together, mix them very well, and put them

them into the Skins. If you find it be too thick, put to it a little Cream. You may boil them near half an Hour, it will make them keep the better.

To make Bologna Sausages.

Take Part of a Leg of Pork or Veal, pick it clean from the Skin or Fat; put to every Pound of lean Meat a Pound of Beef-suet picked from the Skin, shred the Meat and Suet separate and very fine, mix them well together, and add a large Handful of green Sage shred very small; season it with Pepper and Salt, mix it very well, press it down hard in an earthen Pot, and keep it for Use.

When you use them, roll them up with as many Eggs as will make them roll smooth; in rolling them up, make them about the Length of your Fingers, and as thick as two Fingers; fry them in Butter, which must be boiling hot before you can put them in, and keep them rolling about in the Pan. When they are fried through, they are enough.

To make common Sausages.

Chop three Pounds of the best Pork, Fat and Lean together, as fine as possible, but first take care to strip it of its Skin and Gristles; season it with two Tea-spoonfuls of Salt and one of Pepper; to which add three Spoonfuls of Sage shred very fine, and mingle all well together. When your Guts are well cleaned, fill them, or otherwise pot your Ingredients. When you use them, roll them out into what Size you think proper, and fry them as above directed. You may make very agreeable Sausages likewise of Beef, if you chuse it.

To force a Fowl.

Take a good Fowl, pull and draw it, and slit the Skin down the Back; take the Flesh from the Bones, and mince it very well; mix it with a little Beef-suet, shred a Gill of large Oysters, chop a Shalot, a little grated Bread and some sweet Herbs; mix all together, season it with Nutmeg, Pepper and Salt, make it up with Yolks of Eggs, put it on the Bones, and draw the Skin over it; few up the Back, cut off the Legs, and put the Bones as you do a Fowl for boiling; tie up the Fowl in a Cloth; an Hour will boil it. For Sauce, take a few Oysters, shred them, and put them into a little Gravy, with a Lump of Butter, a little Lemon-peel shred, and a little Juice; thicken it with a little Flour, lay the Fowl on the Dish, and pour the Sauce upon it. You may fry a little of the Forcedmeat to lay round. Garnish your Dish with Lemon. You may set it in the Oven if you have Convenience, only rub over it the Yolk of an Egg, and a few Bread-Crumbs.

INSTRUCTIONS *for making* Puddings, Dumplings, Pancakes *and* Fritters *of all Sorts.*

In making your Puddings of all Kinds, the following general Rules are to be observed.

WHEN you boil your Puddings, take particular Care that your Cloth or Bag be perfectly clean, and dipp'd in hot Water, and then too flour'd very well. If it be a Bread-Pudding, tie it loose; but if it be a Batter-Pudding, tie it close; and take care that your Water boils before you put it in. Move your Pudding every now and then, for otherwise it will be apt to stick. If it be a Batter Pudding, mix your Flour well with a little Milk, and then put your Ingredients in by slow Degrees; for by that means it will be free from Lumps, and perfectly smooth. For all other Puddings, when your Eggs are beat, strain them. If you boil them either in Wooden or China Dishes, butter the Inside before you put in your Batter. And as to all baked Puddings, remember to butter your Pan, or Dish, before you put your Pudding into it.

To make Batter Pudding

Take a Pint of Milk, six Eggs, and four Spoonfuls of Flour; put in half a Nutmeg grated, and a little Salt. You must take care your Pudding is not thick. Flour your Cloth well; three Quarters of an Hour will boil it. Serve it up with melted Butter, or with melted Butter, Sugar, and a little Sack.

A Suet Pudding boiled.

Take a Pound of Suet and shred it small; then take a Quart of Milk, four Eggs, one Spoonful of beaten Pepper, or two of beaten Ginger, and a Tea-spoonful of Salt; mix the Flour and Eggs with a Pint of the Milk very thick, and mix the Seasoning with the Remainder of the Milk and the Suet. When you have made your Batter of a good Consistence, boil it above two Hours.

A Plum Pudding boiled.

Cut a Pound of Suet into little Bits, but not shred too fine; take a Pound of Raisins stoned, a Pound of Currants, about eight Eggs, half the Whites, the Crumb of a Penny-Loaf grated very small, half a Nutmeg grated, of beaten Ginger about a Tea-spoonful, a small Quantity of Salt, a Pound of Flour, and a Pint of Milk. First beat your Eggs, then halve the Milk, and beat them together by slow Degrees, then the Suet, Spice, and Fruit, and add to them all as much Milk as will make them of a moderate Consistence. Thus prepared, boil it at least five Hours.

To make an Apple Pudding.

Take half a dozen large Codlings or Pippins, roast them, and take out the Pulp; take eight Eggs, (leave out six of the Whites) half a Pound of fine Powder Sugar, beat your Eggs and Sugar well together, and put to them the Pulp of your Apples, half a Pound of clarified Butter, a little Lemon-peel shred fine, a Handful of Bread-crumbs or Biscuit, four Ounces of candied Orange or Citron, and bake it with a thin Paste under it.

Apple Pudding another Way.

Take four or five Codlings, scald them, and bruise them through a Sieve; put to them a Quarter of a Pound of Biscuits, a little Nutmeg, a Pint of Cream, and sweeten it to your Taste; add ten Eggs, and half the Whites. Bake it.

To make a Bread Pudding.

Take three Gills of Milk; when boiled, take a Penny-Loaf sliced thin, cut off the out Crust, put it into the boiling Milk, let it stand close cover'd till it be cold, and beat it very well till all the Lumps be broke; take five Eggs beat very well, grate in a little Nutmeg, shred some Lemon-peel, and a Quarter of a Pound of Butter or Beef-suet, with as much Sugar as will sweeten it, and Currants as many as you please; let them be well cleaned, so put them into your Dish, and bake or boil it.

To make a Quaking Pudding.

Take eight Eggs, and beat them very well; put to them three Spoonfuls of fine Flour, a little Salt, three Gills of Cream, and boil it with a Stick of Cinnamon and a Blade of Mace. When it is cold, mix it with your Eggs and Flour; butter your Cloth, and do not give it too much Room in your Cloth. About half an Hour will boil it. You must turn it in the boiling, or the Flour will settle. Serve it up with a little melted Butter.

To make a common Quaking Pudding.

Take five Eggs, beat them well with a little Salt, put in three Spoonfuls of fine Flour, take a Pint of new Milk, and beat them well together; then take a Cloth, butter and flour it, but do not give it too much Room in the Cloth. An Hour will boil it, giving it a Turn every now and then at the first putting in, or else the Meal will settle to the Bottom. Having a little plain Butter for Sauce, serve it up.

To make a ground Rice Pudding.

Take a Pound of ground Rice, half cree it in a Quart of Milk; when it is cold, put to it five Eggs well beat, a Gill of Cream, a little Lemon-peel shred fine, half a Nutmeg grated, half a Pound of Butter, and half a Pound of Sugar; mix them well together, put them into your Dish with a little Salt, and bake it with a Puff-paste round your Dish. Have a little Rose-water, Butter and Sugar, to pour over it; you may stick in it candied Lemon or Citron, if you please.

Half of the above Quantity will make a Pudding for a Side-dish.

To make a Marrow Pudding.

Take the Inside of a Penny-Loaf, and cut one Half in thin Slices; take the Marrow of two Bones, half a Pound of Currants well cleaned; shred your Marrow, and sprinkle a little Marrow and Currants over the Dish; if you have not Marrow enough, you may add to it a little Beef-suet shred fine. Take five Eggs, and beat them very well, put to them three Gills of Milk, grate in half a Nutmeg, sweeten it to your Taste, mix all together, pour it over your Pudding, and save a little Marrow to sprinkle over the Top of your Pudding. When you send it to the Oven, lay a Puff-paste round the Edge of the Dish.

To make a Tansey Pudding.

Take an old Penny-Loaf, cut off the out Crust, slice it thin, put to it as much hot Cream as will wet it, six Eggs well beaten, a little shred Lemon-peel; grate in a little Nutmeg, and a little Salt; add to it some Juice of Tansey and Spinage, so tie it up in a Cloth and boil it; it will take an Hour and a Quarter boiling. When you dish it up, stick it with candied Orange, and lay a *Seville* Orange, cut in Quarters, round the Dish; serve it up with melted Butter.

To make a Gooseberry Pudding.

Take a Quart of green Gooseberries, pick, coddle, bruise, and rub them through a Hair Sieve, to take out the Pulp; take six Spoonfuls of Pulp, six Eggs, three Quarters of a Pound of Sugar, half a Pound of clarified Butter, a little Lemon-peel shred fine, a Handful of Bread-crumbs or Biscuit, a Spoonful of Rose or Orange Water; mix these well together, and bake it with a Paste round the Dish. You may add Sweetmeats if you please.

To make a Steak Pudding.

Take some Suet shred small with Flour, and mix it up with cold Water; of this make your Crust; season it with a little Salt, take about two Pounds of Suet to a Quarter of a Peck of Flour. Season your Steaks, whether Beef or Mutton, with Pepper and Salt; make it up in the same Manner as you would an Apple Pudding; tie it up in a Cloth, but let your Water boil before you put it in. If it be but a small Pudding, three Hours will be sufficient; if a large one, five.

To make Suet Dumplings.

Take a Pound of Suet, four Eggs, a Pound of Currants, three Tea-spoonfuls of Ginger, and two of Salt; and to these add a Pint of Milk. First take one Half of the Milk, and mingle it as you would a thick Batter; then put in the Eggs, the Ginger, and the Salt; and then the Remainder of the Milk by slow Degrees, together with the Suet and Currants, and Flour to make it like a light Paste. As soon as your Water boils, make them up in little Rolls, with a small Quantity of Flour; then flat them, and throw them into the boiling Water. Take care to move them gently, that they may not stick to each other. They will be enough in half an Hour, if you keep your Water boiling.

To make a Cuſtard Pudding.

Take a Pint of Cream, mix with it ſix Eggs well beat, two Spoonfuls of Flour, half a Nutmeg grated, a little Salt, and Sugar to your Taſte; butter a Cloth, put it in when the Pot boils, boil it juſt half an Hour, and melt Butter for Sauce.

To make New-College Puddings.

Grate an old Penny-Loaf, put to it a like Quantity of Suet ſhred, a Nutmeg grated, a little Salt and ſome Currants; then beat ſome Eggs in a little Sack and Sugar, mix all together, knead it as ſtiff as for Manchet, and make it up in the Form and Size of a Turkey-Egg; put a little Batter; take a Pound of Butter, put it in a Diſh or Stew-pan, and ſet it over a clear Fire in a Chafing-diſh, and rub your Butter about the Diſh till it is melted; then put your Puddings in, cover the Diſh, and often turn them till they are brown alike. When they are enough, grate ſome Sugar over them, and ſerve them up hot. For a Side-diſh you muſt let the Paſte lay for a Quarter of an Hour before you make up your Puddings.

To make Apple-Dumplings.

Take half a dozen Codlings, or any other good Apples, pare and core them; make a little cold Butter Paſte, and roll it up about the Thickneſs of your Finger, ſo lap round every Apple, and tie them ſingle in a fine Cloth; boil them in a little Salt and Water, and let the Water boil before you put them in; half an Hour will boil them. You muſt have for Sauce a little White-wine and Butter. Grate ſome Sugar round the Diſh, and ſerve them up.

To make plain Fruit Dumplings.

Take as much Flour as you would have Dumplings in Quantity, put to it a Spoonful of Sugar, a little Salt, a little Nutmeg, a Spoonful of light Yeaſt, and half a Pound of Currants well waſh'd and cleaned; ſo knead them to
the

the Stiffness you do a common Dumpling. You must have White-wine, Sugar and Butter for Sauce; you may boil them either in a Cloth or without; so serve them up.

To make Herb Dumplings.

Take a Penny-Loaf, cut off the out Crust, and the rest in Slices; put to it as much hot Milk as will just wet it; take the Yolks and Whites of six Eggs, beat them with two Spoonfuls of Powder Sugar, half a Nutmeg, and a little Salt, so put it to your Bread; take half a Pound of Currants well cleaned, put them to your Eggs, then take a Handful of the mildest Herbs you can get, gather them so equal that the Taste of one be not above the other, wash and chop them very small; put as many of them in as will make a deep Green, (don't put any Parsley amongst them, nor any other strong Herb) so mix them all together, and boil them in a Cloth; make them about the Bigness of middling Apples; about half an Hour will boil them. Put them into your Dish, and have a little candied Orange, White-wine, Butter and Sugar for Sauce; so serve them up.

To make a plain Suet Dumpling.

Take a Pound of Beef Suet shred small, add to it half a Quartern of Flour, then take as much fair Water as will moisten it, to make a thick Paste; then roll them in a little Flour, and put them into the Pot with the Water boiling, and they will be done in half an Hour.

To make fine Pancakes.

Take a Pint of Cream or Milk, eight Eggs, a Nutmeg grated, and a little Salt; then melt a Pound of Butter, and a little Sack, before you stir it. It must be as thick with Flour as ordinary Batter, and fried with Lard. Turn it on the Backside of a Plate; garnish with Orange, and strew Sugar over them.

To make Rice Pancakes.

Take half a Pound of Rice, wash and pick it clean, cree it in fair Water till it be a Jelly; when it is cold, take a Pint of Cream, and the Yolks of four Eggs, beat them very well together, and put them to the Rice, with grated Nutmeg and some Salt; then put in half a Pound of Butter, and as much Flour as will make it thick enough to fry, with as little Butter as you can.

To make Apple Fritters.

Take four Eggs, and beat them very well; put to them four Spoonfuls of fine Flour, a little Milk, about a Quarter of a Pound of Sugar, a little Nutmeg and Salt, so beat them very well together; you must not make them very thin, if you do it will not stick to the Apple. Take a middling Apple and pare it, cut out the Core, and cut the rest in round Slices, about the Thickness of a Shilling; (you may take out the Core after you have cut it with your Thimble) have ready a little Lard in a Stewpan, or any other deep Pan; then take your Apples every Slice single, and dip them into your Batter; let your Lard be very hot, so drop them in; you must keep them turning till enough, and mind that they be not too brown, as you take them out, lay them on a Pewter-Dish before the Fire till you have done; have a little White-wine, Butter and Sugar for the Sauce, grate over them a little Loaf-sugar, and serve them up.

To make Apple Froise.

First cut some Apples in thick Slices, and fry them of a light Brown; take them up and lay them to drain, and keep them as whole as you can; then make the following Batter: Take five Eggs and three Whites, beat them up with Flour and a little Sack; make it the Thickness of a Pancake; pour in a little melted Butter, Nutmeg, and a little Sugar: Melt your Butter, pour in your Batter, and lay a Slice of Apple here and there, and pour more Batter on them; fry them of a fine Brown, then take them up, and ftrew double-refined Sugar over them.

To make Fruit Fritters.

Take a Penny-Loaf, cut off the out Cruft, flice it, put to it as much hot Milk as will wet it, beat five or fix Eggs, put to them a Quarter of a Pound of Currants well cleaned, and a little candied Orange fhred fine; fo mix them well together; drop them with a Spoon into a Stew-pan in clarified Butter; have a little White-wine, Butter and Sugar for your Sauce; put it into a China Bafon, lay your Fritters round, grate a little Sugar over them, and ferve them up.

Rules for making PIES.

To make a Cruft for a Meat Pie.

TAKE one Pound of Flour, and three Quarters of a Pound of Butter, mixed well together, and well beaten with a Rolling-pin. This is fufficient for a common Cruft.

To make a Mutton Pie.

When you have taken off the Skin and Fat of the Infide of a Loin of Mutton, cut the Remainder into Steaks; feafon it to your Palate with Pepper and Salt. When your Cruft is made, fill it with your Meat; after that pour into it as much Water as will near fill the Difh; then put on the Lid, and bake it well.

To make a Beef-Steak Pie.

Take two Pounds of the beft Rump-Steaks, and feafon them with Pepper and Salt, &c. as Mutton Pie.

To make a Mutton Pafty.

Take a Loin of Mutton that is large and fat, and before you bone it, let it hang for five or fix Days. Lay your

your Meat, when boned, four and twenty Hours in about half a Pint of Red Wine, and half a Pint of Rape Vinegar; then take it out of the Pickle, and manage it as you would do a Venison-Pasty. While your Pasty is in the Oven, boil up your Bones in the same Manner, and fill your Pasty with the Liquor, as soon as it comes out of the Oven.

To make a Venison Pasty.

Bone the Neck and the Breast, and season them to your Palate with Pepper and Salt; cut the Breast into three or four Pieces; but, if you can avoid it, cut none of the Fat belonging to the Neck. Lay in the Breast and Neck-end first, and the best of the Neck-end over them, that the Fat may be whole. Let your Crust be made of a rich Puff-paste, very thick on the Sides and also on the Top, and let your Bottom be very good. Cover your Dish first, then lay in your Ingredients; put into them half a Pound of Butter, and above a Quarter of a Pint of Water. Thus prepared, put on your Lid, bake it in a quick Oven, and let it stand there about two Hours. Before it is ready to be taken out, set the Bones of your Venison on the Fire in two Quarts of Water, with three or four Blades of Mace, an Onion, a little Piece of Crust of Bread baked crisp and brown, and a small Quantity of whole Pepper. Let it be close cover'd, and boil softly over a gentle Fire till one Half of your Liquor is wasted, and then strain it off; pour the Remainder into your Pie as soon as it comes from the Oven.

If your Venison happens to be too lean, take the Fat of a Loin of Mutton, and steep it for four and twenty Hours in some Rape Vinegar and Red Wine; then spread it over the Top of your Venison, and cover your Pasty. Though some People imagine that Venison can never be over-baked, and will for that Reason bake it first in a false Crust, yet the Notion is quite wrong; for by such a Practice, the Flavour of the Venison is in some measure, at least, lost and gone. If, however, you are desirous of having it exceedingly tender, you muſt waſh it in warm Milk and Water, and then rub it with clean Cloths till it is perfectly dry. When you have ſo done, rub it all over with the beſt Vinegar, and let it hang in the open Air. You may keep it, thus prepared, for a Fortnight, if you think proper; but then no Moiſture muſt come to it: If you find there does, to prevent its decaying, you muſt dry it well, and then ſtrew Ginger over it.

When you are diſpoſed to make uſe of it, dip it in lukewarm Water, and then wipe it dry again. Let it be baked in a quick Oven. If your Paſty be large, it will require three Hours at leaſt; at which Time it will not only be very tender, but retain its fine Flavour.

N. B. The Shoulder boned, and made as above, with the Mutton-Fat, makes a very agreeable Paſty.

To make an Eel Pie.

Caſe and clean the Eels, ſeaſon them with a little Nutmeg, Pepper and Salt, cut them in long Pieces; you muſt make your Pie with hot Butter Paſte; let it be oval, with a thin Cruſt; lay in your Eels lengthways, and put over them a little freſh Butter; ſo bake them.

Eel Pies are good, and eat very well with Currants; but if you put in Currants, you muſt not uſe any black Pepper, but a little *Jamaica* Pepper.

To make a ſweet Chicken Pie.

Break the Chicken Bones, cut them in little Bits, ſeaſon them lightly with Mace and Salt, take the Yolks of four Eggs boiled hard and quartered, five Artichoke-bottoms, half a Pound of Sun-Raiſins ſtoned, half a Pound of Citron, half a Pound of Lemon, half a Pound of Marrow, a few Forced-meat Balls, and half a Pound of Currants well cleaned, ſo make a light Puff-paſte, but put no Paſte in the Bottom. When it is baked, take a little White-wine, a little Juice either of Orange or Lemon, the Yolk of an Egg well beat, and mix them together, make it hot, and put it into your Pie; when you ſerve

serve it, take the same Ingredients you use for a Lamb or Veal Pie, only leave out the Artichokes.

To make a Pigeon Pie.

Let your Pigeons, in the first place, be very nicely pick'd and clean'd; then season them with Pepper and Salt, either high or low, according to your Palate; and put a good Lump of the best fresh Butter, with Pepper and Salt, into the Bellies of each of them, then cover your Dish with good Puff-paste Crust; in which lay your Birds, so so season'd as aforesaid, with their Necks, Gizzards, Livers, Pinions and Hearts, between them. In the middle lay a large fat Beef-steak, together with the Yolks of hard Eggs, more or less, as you shall judge proper; pour into your Ingredients as much Water as will near fill your Dish; then lay on the Lid or Top-Crust, and bake it well.

To make a Pigeon Pie after the French Fashion.

You must stuff your Pigeons with a very high Forced-meat, and lay a good Quantity of Forced-meat Balls all round the Inside; together with Artichoke Bottoms, Asparagus Tops, Mushrooms, Truffles, and Morels; but season your Ingredients to your Palate, though for the most part they season very high.

To make a Green-Goose Pie.

Bone a Couple of fat Green Geese, and season them pretty high with Salt, Pepper, Nutmeg, and Cloves; and you may, if you like, add a Couple of whole Onions; lay them one on another, fill the Sides, and cover them with Butter and bake them.

To make a Giblet Pie.

Take two Pair of Giblets, that have been carefully cleaned, and put them all into the Saucepan, except the Livers; add to them two Quarts of Water, about two dozen Corns of whole Pepper, three or four Blades of Mace, one large Onion, and a small Bundle of sweet Herbs;

Herbs; let them be covered close, and stew'd very softly till they are perfectly tender; then, when your Crust is duly prepared, cover your Dish with it. Take care to lay a good Rump-steak at the Bottom of your Dish, seasoned to your Palate with Pepper and Salt; after that lay in your Giblets and Livers, and strain the Liquor in which you stew'd them. When you have seasoned them to your Mind, pour it into your Pie, then put the Lid on, and let it stand in the Oven about an Hour and a half.

To make a Duck Pie.

Take two Ducks, and let them be well scalded and cleaned; then cut off the Feet, the Pinions, the Neck and the Head, with the Gizzards, Hearts and Livers, all well cleaned and scalded, as above mentioned; but first pick out all the Fat which you find in the Inside of your Ducks. Lay a good Puff-paste Crust all over your Dish, and put your Materials into it when you have seasoned them to your Liking both inside and out; lay your Giblets, &c. on each side your Ducks. When you have pour'd in as much Water as will near fill your Dish, put on your Lid, and send your Pie to the Oven; but take care it be not over-baked.

To make a Goose Pie.

Half a Peck of Flour will be sufficient to raise the Walls of your Pie with, which must be made just large enough to hold your Goose. In the first place, however, have ready by you a pickled dried Tongue, that has been boil'd so tender as to peel with Ease; cut off the Root, then bone your Goose, and have ready at the same time a large Fowl boned; season your Fowl and your Goose with half a Quarter of an Ounce of Mace beat fine, also a large Tea-spoonful of Pepper beat fine, and three Tea-spoonfuls of Salt, all well mingled together; then lay your Fowl into your Goose, and your Tongue into your Fowl, and your Goose in the very same Form as if it were whole; put about half a Pound of the best Butter upon the Top, and

and then lay on your Lid. This is a very good Pie, either hot or cold, and will keep some considerable Time.

To make Minced Pie with Calves-Feet.

Take two or three Calves-Feet, and boil them as you would do for eating; take out the long Bones, shred them very fine, put to them double their Weight of Beef-suet shred fine, and about a Pound of Currants well cleaned, a Quarter of a Pound of candied Orange and Citron cut in small Pieces, half a Pound of Sugar, a little Salt, a Quarter of a Pound of Mace, and a large Nutmeg; beat them together, put in a little Juice of Lemon or Verjuice to your Taste, a Glass of Mountain Wine or Sack, which you please, and mix all together; bake them in Puff-paste.

To make a Calf's-Head Pie.

Take a Calf's-Head and clean it, boil it as you would do for hashing; when it is cold, cut it in thin Slices, and season it with a little black Pepper, Nutmeg and Salt, a few shred Capers, a few Oysters and Cockles, two or three Mushrooms, and green Lemon-peel; mix them all well together, and put them into your Pie. It must be a standing Pie, baked in a flat Pewter Dish, with a Rim of Puff-paste round the Edge. When you have fill'd the Pie with the Meat, lay on Forced-meat Balls, and the Yolks of some hard Eggs, put in a little small Gravy and Butter. When it comes from the Oven, take off the Lid, put into it a little White-wine to your Taste, and shake up the Pie; so serve it up without a Lid.

To make a Calf's-Foot Pie.

Take two or three Calves-Feet, according as you would have your Pie in Bigness, boil and bone them as you would do for Eating, and when cold, cut them in thin Slices; take about three Quarters of a Pound of Beef-suet shred fine, half a Pound of Raisins stoned, half a Pound of cleaned Currants, a little Mace and Nutmeg, green Lemon or Orange; mix all together, and put them into a Dish,

Dish, make a good Puff-paste, but let there be no Paste at the Bottom of the Dish. When it is baked, take off the Lid, and squeeze in a little Lemon or Verjuice; cut the Lid in Sippets, and lay round.

To make a Woodcock Pie.

Take three or four Brace of Woodcocks, according as you would have the Pie in Bigness, dress and skewer them as you would do for Roasting; draw them, and season the Inside with a little Pepper, Salt, and Mace, but do not wash them; put the Trails into the Belly again, but nothing else; for there is something in them that gives them a more bitterish Taste in the Baking, than in the Roasting. When you put them into your Dish, lay them with the Breast downwards, beat them upon the Breast as flat as you can; you must season them on the Outside as you do the Inside. Bake them in Puff-paste, but lay none in the Bottom of your Dish; put to them a Gill of Gravy, and a little Butter. You must be careful your Pie be not too much baked. When you serve it up, take off the Lid, and turn the Woodcocks with the Breast upwards. You may bake Partridges the same Way.

To make a Rabbet Pie.

Cut young Rabbets in pieces, and fry them in Lard with a little Flour; season them with Salt, Pepper, Nutmeg, sweet Herbs, and Chibbols, adding a little Broth. When they are cold, put them into your Pie, adding some Morels, Truffles, and pounded Lard; lay on the Lid, set it in the Oven, and let it stand for an Hour and half; when it is about half baked, pour in the Sauce in which the Rabbets were fried; and just before you serve it up to Table, squeeze in some Juice of *Seville* Orange.

To make a Hare Pie.

Having cut the Hare into pieces, break the Bones, and lay them in the Pie; lay on sliced Lemon, Balls, and Butter, and close it with the Yolks of hard Eggs.

To make a Turbot-Head Pie.

Take a middling Turbot-Head, pretty well cut off, wash it clean, take out the Gills, season it pretty well with Mace, Pepper, and Salt, so put it into a deep Dish, with half a Pound of Butter; cover it with light Puff-paste, but lay none in the Bottom; when it is baked, take out the Liquor and the Butter that it was baked in; put it into a Saucepan, with a Lump of fresh Butter and Flour to thicken it, with an Anchovy and a Glass of White-wine, so pour it into your Pie again over the Fish. You may lay round half a dozen Yolks of Eggs at an equal Distance. When you have cut off the Lid, lay it in Sippets round your Dish, and serve it up.

To make a Turkey Pie.

Take a Turkey and bone it, season it with savoury Spice, and lay it in the Pie, with two Capons cut in pieces to fill up the Corners: The Crust to be made in the same Manner as you would do for a Goose Pie.

To make a Trout Pie.

Having cleaned and scalded them, lard them with Pieces of Silver Eel roll'd up in Spice, and sweet Herbs and Bay Leaves powder'd; lay between them, and on them, the Bottoms of Artichokes sliced, Oysters, Mushrooms, Capers, and sliced Lemon; lay on Butter, and close the Pie.

A Pork Pie.

First skin your Pork, then cut it into Steaks; season it pretty well with Salt, Nutmeg sliced, and beaten Pepper; put in some Pippins cut in small Pieces, as many as you think convenient, and sweeten with Sugar to your Palate; put in half a Pint of White-wine; lay Butter all over it, close up your Pie, and set it in the Oven.

Pork Pie to be eaten cold.

Take a Loin of Pork, bone it, and cut Part of it into Collops; take also as many Collops of Veal of the same Size,

Size, and beat them both with the Back of a Cleaver; feafon the Pork with Salt, Pepper, minced Sage, and the Yolks of hard Eggs; feafon your Veal with Cloves, Mace, Nutmeg, Thyme minced, and the Yolks of hard Eggs; then lay in your Difh a Layer of Pork and a Layer of Veal, till you have laid all your Meat in; then clofe up your Pie, and liquor it with Saffron-Water, or the Yolks of Eggs. When it is baked, fill it with clarified Butter. Remember to let your firft and laft Layer be Pork; bake it, and fet it by for Ufe.

To make a very good Pie.

Lay fome Puff-pafte round the Brims of your Difh; then lay a Layer of Bifcuit, and a Layer of Marrow and Butter, then a Layer of all Sorts of wet Sweet-meats, or as many as you can have, and do fo till your Difh is full; then boil a Quart of Cream, and thicken it with two Eggs, a little Rofe-water and Sugar; put this to the reft, and bake.

A Bride Pie.

Parboil Cocks-combs, and ftew Veal Sweetbreads and Lamb-ftones; cut them into thin Slices; alfo blanch Ox-palates, and cut them into Slices; to thefe put a Pint of Oyfters, fome Slices of interlarded Bacon, a few Broom-buds pickled, a few Chefnuts roafted and blanched, a Handful of Pine-kernels and fome Dates fliced; feafon thefe with Salt and Nutmeg, and whole Mace; fill your Pie with thefe, lay Slices of Butter over them, clofe it up, and bake it. When it comes out of the Oven, cut up the Lid, and having beaten up Butter with the Yolks of three or four Eggs, fome Wine, and the Juice of a Lemon, well fhaken together, pour this into your Pie.

A Tench Pie.

Having made your Cruft, lay on it a Layer of Butter, then fcatter in grated Nutmeg, Cinnamon, and Mace; then lay in half a dozen Tench, lay Butter over them, and a few blue Currants; pour in a Quarter of a Pint of Claret,

Claret, and let them be well baked. When it comes out of the Oven, put in melted Butter, duſt it over with ſome fine Sugar, and ſerve it up.

Instructions *for making* Fruit-Pies, Tarts, Cheeſecakes *and* Cuſtards.

To make a Paſte for a Fruit Pie.

TAKE half a Pound of Flour, half a Pound of Butter, and half a Pound of Sugar; then mix your Ingredients well all together, beat them well with a Rolling-pin, and when rolled out thin, it is ready for your Purpoſe.

A good Paſte for Tarts.

Take a Pint of Flour, and rub a Quarter of a Pound of Butter into it; beat two Eggs, with a Spoonful of double-refined Sugar, and two or three Spoonfuls of Cream to make it into Paſte; work it as little as you can, roll it out thin, butter your Tins, duſt on ſome Flour, then lay in your Paſte, and do not fill them too full.

To make Paſte for Tarts.

Take the Yolks of five or ſix Eggs, juſt as you would have Paſte in Quantity; to the Yolks of ſix Eggs put a Pound of Butter; work the Butter with your Hand till it take up all the Eggs; then take ſome *London* Flour, and work it with your Butter till it comes to a Paſte; put in about two Spoonfuls of Loaf-Sugar beat and ſifted, and about half a Gill of Water. When you have wrought it well together, it is fit for Uſe.

This is Paſte that ſeldom runs, if it be even roll'd. Roll it thin, but let your Lids be thinner than your Bottoms. When you have made your Tarts, prick them over with a Pin, to keep them from bliſtering. When you are going to put them into the Oven, wet them over with a
Feather

Feather dipt in fair Water, and grate over them a little double-refined Loaf-Sugar, it will ice them; but do not let them be baked in a hot Oven.

A short Paste for Tarts.

Take a Pound of Wheat Flour, and rub it very small, three Quarters of a Pound of Butter, rub it as small as the Flour; put to it three Spoonfuls of Loaf-Sugar beat and sifted; take the Yolks of four Eggs, and beat them very well; put to them a Spoonful or two of Rose-water, and work them into a Paste; then roll them thin, and ice them over as you did the other, if you please, and bake them in a slow Oven.

To make a Shell-Paste.

Take half a Pound of fine Flour, and a Quarter of a Pound of Butter, the Yolks of four Eggs and one White, two Ounces of Sugar finely sifted; mix all these together with a little Water, and roll it very thin till you can see through it. When you lid your Tarts, prick them, to keep them from blistering; be sure to roll them even, and when you bake them ice them.

To make a Dripping Crust.

Boil a Pound and a half of Beef Dripping in Water, strain it, and let it stand till it be cold; then take off the hard Fat, which, when you have scraped well, must be boiled four or five times successively. Let this be afterwards work'd up well into three Pounds of Flour as fine as possible, and then make it up into Paste with cold Water. This Crust will eat very agreeably, and please the nicest Palate.

To make a Crust for Custards.

To half a Pound of Flour add six Ounces of Butter, three Spoonfuls of Cream, and the Yolks of two Eggs; mix them well together, and let them stand for about a Quarter of an Hour; after that work it up and down well, and roll it as thin as you please.

To make an Apple Pie.

Scald about a dozen Apples very tender, and take off the Skin; then take the Pap of them, and put to it twelve Eggs, but six Whites; beat them very well, and take the Crumb of a Penny-Loaf grated, and a Nutmeg grated; sugar it to your Taste, and put in a Quarter of a Pound of Butter melted; mix all these together, and bake them in a Dish; butter your Dish, and take care that your Oven is not too hot.

To make an Apple Pie another Way.

Take a Quarter of a Peck of large Apples, pare them, and cut them into thin Slices; then put a Pound of Powder Sugar, with a little Water, and lay on your Crust, made after the Directions given how *to make a Paste for a Fruit Pie* You may cut up the Top, and put in some Butter, if it is to be eaten hot; if not, it will be as good without the Butter.

You may make Gooseberry, Currant, Cherry, Damson, and all Sorts of Fruit Pies for a Family, by the same Rule.

To make Tarts of divers Kinds

If you propose to bake them in Patty-pans, first butter them well, and then put a thin Crust all over them, in order to your taking them out with the greater Ease; but if you make use of either Glass or China Dishes, add no Crust but the top one. Strew a proper Quantity of fine Sugar at the Bottom in the first place, and after that lay in your Fruit of what Sort soever, as you think most proper, and strew the like Quantity of the same Sugar over them; then put your Lid on, and let them be baked in a slack Oven. Observe, however, that Minced Pies must always be baked in Patty-pans, on account of taking them out with the greater Ease, as above hinted, and Puff-paste is the most proper for them. If you make Tarts of Apples, Pears, Apricots, &c. the beaten Crust is looked upon as the most proper; but that is submitted to your own particular Fancy

I To

To make Apple or Pear Tart.

Pare them first; then cut them into Quarters, and take the Cores out; in the next place, cut each Quarter across again; throw them, so prepared, into a Saucepan with no more Water in it than what will just cover your Fruit; let them simmer over a slow Fire till they are perfectly tender: However, before you set your Fruit on the Fire, take care to put a good large Piece of Lemon-peel into your Water. Have your Patty-pans in Readiness, and strew fine Sugar at the Bottom; then lay in your Fruit, and cover them with as much of the same Sugar as you think convenient. Over each Tart pour a Tea-spoonful of Lemon-Juice, and three Spoonfuls of the Liquor in which they were boiled. Then lay your Lid over them, and put them into a slack Oven. Observe, If your Tarts be made of Apricots, you must use no Lemon-Juice, which is the only material Difference in the Manner of making them. Observe likewise, with respect to preserved Tarts only, lay in your preserved Fruit, and put a very thin Crust over them, and bake them as short a Time as possible.

To make Orange Tart.

Take two or three *Seville* Oranges, and boil them; shift them in the boiling to take out the Bitter; cut them in two, take out the Oranges, and cut them in Slices; they must be baked in crisp Paste. When you fill the Patty-pans, lay in a Layer of Oranges and a Layer of Sugar, (a Pound will sweeten a dozen of small Tins, if you do not put in too much Orange) bake them in a slow Oven, and ice them over.

To make a Sweet-meat Tart.

Make a little Shell-paste, roll it, and line your Tins; prick them in the Inside, and so bake them; then you may serve them up with any Sort of Sweet-meats, what you please. You may have a different Sort every Day, do but keep your Shells baked by you.

To make Cheese-cakes.

Take a Gallon of new Milk, make of it a tender Curd, squeeze the Whey from it, put it into a Bason, and break three Quarters of a Pound of Butter into the Curd, then with a clean Hand work the Butter and Curd together till all the Butter be melted, and rub it in a Hair-sieve with the back of a Spoon till all be through; then take six Eggs, beat them with a few Spoonfuls of Rose-water or Sack, put it into your Curd, with half a Pound of fine Sugar and a Nutmeg grated; mix them all together, with a little Salt, and some Currants and Almonds; then make up your Paste of fine Flour, with cold Butter and a little Sugar; roll your Paste very thin, fill your Tins with the Curd, and set them in an Oven. When they are almost enough, take them out, then take a Quarter of a Pound of Butter, with a little Rose-water, and Part of half a Pound of Sugar; let it stand on the Coals till all the Butter be melted, then pour into each Cake some of it, set them in the Oven again till they be brown; so keep them for Use.

To make common Curd Cheese-cakes.

Take a Pennyworth of Curds, mix them with a little Cream, beat four Eggs, put to them six Ounces of clarified Butter, a Quarter of a Pound of Sugar, half a Pound of Currants well wash'd, and a little Lemon-peel shred, a little Nutmeg, a Spoonful of Rose-water or Brandy, which you please, and a little Salt; mix all together, and bake them in small Patty-pans.

To make Cheese-cakes without Currants.

Take five Quarts of new Milk, and run it to a tender Curd, then hang it in a Cloth to drain; rub into it a Pound of Butter that is well washed in Rose-water, put to it the Yolks of seven or eight Eggs, and two of the Whites; season it with Cinnamon, Nutmeg, and Sugar.

To make a Tanfey.

Take a Pint of Cream, some Biscuits without Seeds, two or three Spoonfuls of fine Flour, nine Eggs, leaving out two of the Whites, some Nutmeg, and Orange-flower Water, a little Juice of Tansey and Spinage; put it into a Pan till it be pretty thick, then fry or bake it; if fried, take care that you do not let it be too brown. Garnish your Dish with Orange and Sugar, and serve it up.

To make a Cherry Tart.

Get two Pounds of Cherries, stone, bruise, and stamp them; then boil up their Juice with Sugar; then stone four Pounds more of Cherries, and put them into your Tart with the Cherry Syrup, bake the Tart, ice it, and serve it up hot.

To make a Gooseberry Tart.

Prepare the Crust for your Patty-pans, sheet the Bottoms, and strew them over with Powder-Sugar; then take green Gooseberries, and fill your Tarts with them, laying them in one by one, a Layer of Gooseberries and a Layer of Sugar, so close your Tarts, and bake them in a quick Oven, and they will be very clear and green.

To make Lemon Cheese-cakes.

Boil the Peel of two large Lemons very tender, then throw them into a Mortar, and pound them well with near half a Pound of double-refined Sugar; then take half a dozen Eggs, and half a Pound of the best fresh Butter you can get; pound all these Materials till they are well mingled together, have a Puff-paste in your Patty-pans ready for Use, and when you have filled them half full, send them to the Oven.

N. B. Orange Cheese-cakes are made the same Way with this small Difference only, that your Peels must be boiled in several Waters, for otherwise your Cheese-cakes will be bitter.

To make Marrow Tarts

To a Quart of Cream put the Yolks of twelve Eggs, half a Pound of Sugar, some beaten Mace and Cinnamon, a little Salt, and some Sack; set it on the Fire, with half a Pound of Biscuit, as much Marrow, a little Orange-peel and Lemon-peel; stir it on the Fire till it becomes thick, and when it is cold put it into a Dish with good Puff-paste, then bake it gently in a slow Oven.

To make Almond Puffs.

Take a Pound of Almonds blanched, and beat them with Orange-flower Water; then take a Pound of Sugar, and boil them almost to a Candy-height; put in your Almonds, and stir them on the Fire, keep stirring them till they be cold; beat them a Quarter of an Hour in a Mortar, put to them a Pound of Sugar sifted, and a little Lemon-peel grated, make it into a Paste with the Whites of three Eggs, and beat them into a Froth, more or less, as you think proper; bake them in an Oven almost cold, and keep them for Use.

To make baked Custards.

Boil in the first place a Pint of Cream, with a small Quantity of Mace and Cinnamon in it; and as soon as it is cold, take four Eggs, leaving out one half of the Whites, a small Quantity of Rose and Orange-flower Water mixed with Sack, and as much double-refined Sugar and Nutmeg as will suit your Palate. Mix your Ingredients well together before you send them to the Oven, and bake them in China Cups.

To make Almond Custards.

Take a Quarter of a Pound of Almonds that have been beaten fine, with two Spoonfuls of Rose-water, and put them into a Pint of Cream; then add to it such a Quantity of double refined Sugar as will sweeten it to your Palate. In the next place, beat up the Yolks of four Eggs, and set them, when mixed with your other Ingredients, over the Fire, stirring them all the Time one Way only till they are of a proper Consistence, and then pour out into little Cups; or you may bake them in small China Cups.

To make common Custards.

Sweeten a Quart of new Milk with Loaf-Sugar, according to your Taste, and put into it some grated Nutmeg; then beat up eight Eggs very well, leaving out four of the Whites, and stir them amongst your Milk; then bake them either in small China Basons, or put the whole into one deep Dish. Set the Dish in hot boiling Water, that will rise about half-way. If you think proper, you may add a little Rose-water before you serve it up.

To make Orange Butter.

Beat the Yolks of ten Eggs very well, and add to them half a Pint of Rhenish, six Ounces of double-refined Sugar, and the Juice of three sweet Oranges; set your Ingredients on the Fire, and continue stirring them one way only, till they come to a Consistence; then take them off and stir them; put into them a Lump of Butter about the Bigness of a large Walnut.

INSTRUCTIONS *for making various Kinds of* Cakes, Gingerbread, Biscuits, Macaroons, Wigs, *and* Buns.

To make Gingerbread.

TAKE two Ounces of Ginger, a Quarter of an Ounce each of Nutmegs, Cloves, and Mace, all beaten very fine, and mix them with three Quarts of fine Flour; add three Quarters of a Pound of double-refined Sugar, and two Pounds of Treacle; set them over the Fire, but don't let them boil; mix into the Treacle three Quarters of a Pound of melted Butter, and some Lemon and Orange peel candied and shred small. When all your Ingre-

Ingredients have been well mixed together, set them in a quick Oven, and let them stand for an Hour only, and your Bread will be sufficiently baked.

To make red Gingerbread.

Take a Quart and a Gill of Red Wine, a Gill and a half of Brandy, seven or eight Manchets, according to the Size the Bread is; grate them, (the Crust must be dried, beat and sifted) three Pounds and a half of Sugar beat and sifted, two Ounces of Cinnamon, a Pound of Almonds blanched and beat with Rose-water; put the Bread into the Liquor by degrees, stirring it all the Time; when the Bread is all well mixed, take it off the Fire. You must put the Sugar, Spices, and Almonds into it; when it is cold, print it; keep some of the Spice to dust the Prints with.

To make white Gingerbread.

Take a little Gum-Dragon, lay it in Rose-water all Night, then take a Pound of Jordan Almonds blanched, with a little of the Gum-water, a Pound of double-refined Sugar beat and sifted, an Ounce of Cinnamon beat, with a little Rose-water; work it into a Paste, and print it, then set it in a Stove to dry.

To make Icing for a Cake.

Take two Pounds of double-refined Sugar, beat it, and sift it through a fine Sieve; put to it a Spoonful of fine Starch, a Pennyworth of Gum-Arabic; beat them well together: Take the Whites of four or five Eggs, beat them well, and put to them a Spoonful of Rose-water or Orange-flower-water, a Spoonful of Juice of Lemon; beat them with the Whites of your Eggs, and put in a little to your Sugar till you wet it, then beat them for two Hours while your Cake is baking. If you make it too thin, it will run; when you lay it on your Cake, you must lay it on a Knife. If you would have the Icing very thick, you must add a little more Sugar; wipe off the loose Currants

before

before you put on the Icing, and put it into the Oven to harden the Icing.

To make a Plum Cake.

Take five Pounds of Flour dried and cold, mix with it an Ounce of Mace, half an Ounce of Cinnamon, a Quarter of an Ounce of Nutmegs, half a Quarter of an Ounce of Lemon-peel grated, and a Pound of fine Sugar; take fifteen Eggs, leaving out seven of the Whites, beat your Eggs with half a Gill of Brandy or Sack, a little Orange-Flower or Rose-Water; then put to your Eggs near a Quart of Cream, and three Pounds of Butter, let your Butter melt in the Cream, so let it stand till Milk-warm; then skim off all the Butter, and most of the Milk, and mix to it your Eggs and Yeast; make a Hole in the Middle of your Flour, and put in your Yeast, sprinkle at the Top a little Flour; then mix with it a little Salt, six Pounds of Currants well wash'd, clean'd, dry'd, pick'd, and plump'd by the Fire, a Pound of the best Raisins stoned, and beat them all together till they leave the Bowl; put in a Pound of candy'd Orange, and half a Pound of Citron cut in long Pieces; then butter the Garth, and fill it full; bake it in a quick Oven, against it be enough have an Icing ready.

To make a Carraway Cake.

Take eighteen Eggs, leave out Half of the Whites, and beat them; take two Pounds of Butter, wash the Butter clear from Milk and Salt; put to it a little Rose-Water, and wash your Butter very well with your Hands till it take up all the Eggs, then mix them in half a Jack of Brandy and Sack; grate into your Eggs a Lemon-Rind; put in by Degrees (a Spoonful at a Time) two Pounds of fine Flour, a Pound and a Half of Loaf Sugar, that is sifted and dry; when you have mixed them very well with your Hands, take a Thible, and beat it very well for Half an Hour, till it looks very white, then mix to it a few Seeds, six Ounces of Carraway

The Young Woman's best Companion. 93

Comfits, and half a Pound of Citron and candied Orange, then beat it well, butter your Garth, and put it in a quick Oven.

To make Cakes to keep all the Year.

Have in readiness a Pound and four Ounces of Flour, well dried; take a Pound of fresh Butter, work it with a Pound of white Sugar till it creams, three Spoonfuls of Sack, and the Rind of an Orange; boil it till it is not bitter, and beat it with Sugar; work these together, then clean your Hands, and grate a Nutmeg into your Flour; put in three Eggs and two Whites; mix them well, then with a Paste-pin, or Thible, stir in your Flour to the Butter, make them up into little Cakes, wet the Top with Sack, and strew on fine Sugar; bake them on butter'd Papers well floured, but not too much; you may add a Pound of Currants washed and warmed.

To make Shrewsbury *Cakes.*

Take two Pounds of fine Flour, put to it a Pound and a Quarter of fine Sugar sifted, grate in a Nutmeg, beat in three Whites of Eggs and two Yolks, with a little Rose-water, and so knead your Paste with it; let it lie an Hour, then make it up into Cakes; prick them, and lay them on Papers; wet them with a Feather dipp'd in Rose-water, and grate over them a little fine Sugar. Bake them in a slow Oven, either on Tins or Paper.

To make a fine Cake.

Take five Pounds of fine Flour dried, and keep it warm; four Pounds of Loaf-sugar pounded, sifted, and warmed; five Pounds of Currants well cleaned and warm'd before the Fire; a Pound and half of Almonds blanched, beat, dried, slit, and kept warm; five Pounds of good Butter, well washed and beat from the Water; then work it an Hour and a half till it comes to a fine Cream; put to the Butter all the Sugar, and work it up, and then the Flour; put in a Pint of Brandy, then all the Whites and
Yolks

Yolks of the Eggs; mix all the Currants and Almonds with the rest. There must be four Pounds of Eggs in Weight in the Shells, the Yolks and Whites beat and separated, the Whites beat to a Froth; you must not cease beating till they are beat to a Curd, to prevent oiling. To the Quantity of a Cake put a Pound and a half of Orange-peel and Citron, shred, without Plums, and half a Pound of Carraway Seeds. It will require four Hours baking, and the Oven must be as hot as for Bread; but let it be well slaked when it has remained an Hour in the Oven, and stop it up close; you may ice it if you please.

To make a Seed Cake.

Take a Quartern of fine Flour, well dried before the Fire; when it is cold, rub in a Pound of Butter. Take three Quarters of a Pound of Carraway Comfits, six Spoonfuls of new Yeast, six Spoonfuls of Cream, the Yolks of six Eggs and two Whites, and a little Sack: Mix all these together in a very light Paste, set it before the Fire till it rises, and so bake it in a Tin.

To make an ordinary Plum Cake.

Take a Pound of Flour well dried before the Fire, a Pound of Currants, two Pennyworth of Mace and Cloves, two Eggs, four Spoonfuls of good new Yeast, half a Pound of Butter, half a Pint of Cream; melt the Butter, warm the Cream, and mix all together in a very light Paste; butter your Tin before you put it in; an Hour will bake it.

To make Breakfast Cakes.

Take a Pound of Currants well wash'd, (rub them in a Cloth till dry) a Pound of Flour dried before the Fire; take three Eggs, leave out one of the Whites, four Spoonfuls of new Yeast, four Spoonfuls of Sack, or two of Brandy. Beat the Yeast and Eggs well together; then take a Gill of Cream, and something above a Quarter of a Pound of Butter; set them on the Fire, and stir them till the Butter be melted, but do not let them boil; grate a large Nutmeg

Nutmeg into the Flour with Currants, and five Spoonfuls of Sugar; mix all together, beat it with your Hand till it leaves the Bowl; then flour the Tins you put your Paste in, and let them stand a little to rise; then bake them an Hour and a Quarter.

To make Macaroons.

Take a Pound of blanch'd Almonds and beat them; put some Rose-water in while beating; (they must not be beaten too small) mix them with the Whites of five Eggs, a Pound of Sugar finely beaten and sifted, and a Handful of Flour; mix all these very well together, lay them on Wafers, and bake them in a very temperate Oven, (it must not be so hot as for Manchet) then they are fit for Use.

To make Wigs.

Take two Pounds of Flour, a Pound of Butter, a Pint of Cream, four Eggs, (leaving out two of the Whites) and two Spoonfuls of Yeast; set them to rise a little; when they are mixed, add half a Pound of Sugar, half a Pound of Carraway Comfits; make them up with Sugar, and bake them in a Dripping-pan.

To make Portugal Cakes.

Take a Pound of Flour, a Pound of Butter, a Pound of Sugar, a Pound of Currants well cleaned, and a Nutmeg grated; take half of the Flour, and mix it with Sugar and Nutmeg, melt the Butter, and put into it the Yolks of eight Eggs very well beat, and only four of the Whites; and as the Froth rises put it into the Flour, and so do till all is in: Then beat it together, still strewing some of the other Half of the Flour, and then beat it till all the Flour be in; then butter the Pans and fill them, but do not bake them too much. You may ice them if you please, or you may strew Carraway Comfits of all Sorts on them when they go into the Oven. The Currants must be plump'd in warm Water, and dried before the Fire, then put them into your Cakes.

To make a Biscuit Cake.

Take a Pound of *London* Flour dried before the Fire, a Pound of Loaf-sugar beaten and sifted; beat nine Eggs and a Spoonful or two of Rose-water with the Sugar for two Hours, then put them to your Flour, and mix them well together; put in an Ounce of Carraway Seeds, then put it into your Tin, and bake it an Hour and a half in a pretty quick Oven.

To make Cracknels.

Take half a Pound of fine Flour, half a Pound of Sugar, two Ounces of Butter, two Eggs, and a few Carraway Seeds; (you must beat and sift the Sugar) then put it to your Flour, and work it to a Paste; roll them as thin as you can, and cut them out with Queen-Cake Tins; lay them on Papers, and bake them in a slow Oven. They are proper to eat with Chocolate.

To make Paste Royal for Patty-pans.

Work up a Pound of Flour with half a Pound of Butter, two Ounces of fine Sugar, and Eggs.

INSTRUCTIONS *for making* Creams, Jellies, Syllabubs, &c.

To make Chocolate Cream.

TAKE four Ounces of Chocolate, more or less, according as you would have your Dish in Bigness, grate it, and boil it in a Pint of Cream, then mill it very well with a Chocolate-stick; take the Yolks of two Eggs, and beat them very well, leaving out the Strain; put to them three or four Spoonfuls of Cream, mix them all together; set it on the Fire, and keep it stirring till it thickens, but do not let it boil. You must sweeten it to your Taste, and keep stirring it till it be cold; so put it into your Glasses, or China Dishes, which you please.

To make Cream Curds.

Take a Gallon of Water, put to it a Quart of new Milk, a little Salt, a Pint of sweet Cream, and eight Eggs, leaving out half of the Whites and Strains; beat them very well, put to them a Pint of sour Cream, mix them very well together, and when your Pan is just at boiling, (but it must not boil) put in the sour Cream and your Eggs, stir it about, and keep it from settling to the Bottom; let it stand till it begins to rise up, then have a little fair Water, and, as they rise, keep putting it in till they are well risen, then take them off the Fire, and let them stand a little to sadden; have ready a Sieve with a clean Cloth over it, and take up the Curds with a Ladder or Egg-Slice, which you have. You must always make them the Night before you use them. This Quantity will make a large Dish, if your Cream be good. If you think your Curds be too thick, mix with them two or three Spoonfuls of good Cream, so lay them upon a China Dish in Lumps, and serve them up.

To make Apple Cream.

Take half a dozen large Apples, Codlins, or any other Apples that will be soft, and coddle them; when they are cold, take out the Pulp; then take the Whites of four or five Eggs, (leaving out the Strains) three Quarters of a Pound of double-refined Sugar beat and sifted, a Spoonful or two of Rose-water, and grate in a little Lemon-peel, and so beat all together for an Hour, till it be white; then lay it on a China Dish, so serve it up.

To make Raspberry Cream.

Take Raspberries, bruise them, put them into a Pan on a quick Fire till the Juice be dried up; then take the same Weight of Sugar as you have of Raspberries, and let them on a slow Fire; let them boil till they are pretty stiff; make them into Cakes, and dry them near the Fire, or in the Sun.

K

To make Strawberry and Raspberry Fool.

Take a Pint of Raspberries, squeeze and strain the Juice with a Spoonful of Orange-Water, put to the Juice six Ounces of fine Sugar, and boil it over the Fire; then take a Pint of Cream and boil it, mix them together, and heat them over the Fire, but not to boil; if it do, it will curdle; stir it till it be cold, put it into your Bason, and keep it for Use.

To make Gooseberry Cream.

Take a Quart of Gooseberries; pick, coddle, and bruise them very well in a Marble Mortar or wooden Bowl, and rub them with the Back of a Spoon through a Hair-sieve, till you take out all the Pulp from the Seeds; take a Pint of thick Cream, mix it well among your Pulp, grate in some Lemon-peel, and sweeten it to your Taste; serve it up either in a China Dish, or an earthen one.

To make a Dish of Mull'd Milk.

Boil a Quart of new Milk with a Stick of Cinnamon, then put to it a Pint of Cream, and let them have one Boil together; take eight Eggs, leave out half of the Whites and all the Strains, beat them very well, put to them a Gill of Milk, mix all together, and set it over a slow Fire; stir it till it begins to thicken like Custard, sweeten it to your Taste, and grate in half a Nutmeg; then put it into your Dish with a Toast of Wheat Bread. This is proper for a Supper.

To make Leatch.

Take two Ounces of Isinglass, and break it into Bits, put it into hot Water, then put half a Pint of new Milk into the Pan with the Isinglass, set it on the Fire to boil, and put into it three or four Sticks of good Cinnamon, two Blades of Mace, a Nutmeg quarter'd, and two or three Cloves; boil it till the Isinglass be dissolved, run it through a Hair-sieve into a large Pan, then put to it a Quart of Cream sweeten'd to your Taste with Loaf-sugar,

and

and boil them a while together; take a Quarter of a Pound of blanch'd Almonds beaten in Rose-Water, and strain out all the Juice of them into the Cream on the Fire, and warm it, then take it off and stir it well together. When it has cooled a little, take a broad shallow Dish, and put it into it through a Hair-sieve; when it is cold, cut it in long Pieces, and lay it across till you have a pretty large Dish; so serve it up. Sometimes a less Quantity of Isinglass will do, according to the Goodness. Let it be the whitest and clearest you can get. You must make it the Day before you want it for Use.

To make white Lemon Cream.

Take a Gill of Spring-Water, and a Pound of fine Sugar, set it over the Fire till the Sugar be dissolved; then put the Juice of four good Lemons to your Sugar and Water, the Whites of four Eggs well beat; set it on the Fire again, and keep it stirring one Way till it just simmers and does not boil; strain it through a fine Cloth, then put it on the Fire again, adding to it a Spoonful of Orange-flower-Water; stir it till it thickens on a slow Fire, then strain it into Basons or Glasses for your Use. Do not let it boil; if you do, it will curdle.

To make Cream Cheese.

Take three Quarts of new Milk, one Quart of Cream, a Spoonful of Earning, put them together, let it stand till it comes to the Hardness of a strong Jelly; then put it into the Mould, shifting it often into dry Cloths, lay the Weight of three Pounds upon it, and about two Hours after you may lay six or seven Pounds more; turn it often into dry Cloths till Night, then take the Weight off, and let it lie in the Mould without Weight and Cloth till Morning, and when it is so dry that it doth not wet a Cloth, keep it in Greens till fit for Use. If you please, you may put a little Salt into it.

To make Orange Cream.

Squeeze as many *Seville* Oranges into a Bason as will produce you about a Pint of Liquor, and add thereto the Yolks of half a dozen Eggs, with two Thirds of the Whites only. When you have beaten them well together, into this beat and sift a sufficient Quantity of the best Loaf-sugar; then put your Ingredients into a Silver Saucepan, and set them over a gentle Fire; put in the Peel of half an Orange only, and keep stirring it all the Time one Way. When it is very hot, (for it must not boil) take out the Orange-peel, and pour out your Cream into China Dishes, or little Glasses.

To make Barley Cream.

Boil such a Quantity of Pearl Barley as you think proper to use, in Milk and Water, until it is perfectly tender; then, having strained your Liquor from it, put your Barley into a Quart of Cream, set them over the Fire, and give them a gentle Boil; then beat up with a Spoonful of fine Flour, and two Spoonfuls of Rose or Orange-flower Water, the Yolk of one Egg only, the Whites of five or six; after that, take your Cream off the Fire, and mix your Eggs with it gradually; then set your Ingredients once more over the Fire, that they may thicken. When you have sweetened the Whole to your Palate, pour it into small Basons, but do not serve it up to Table till it is perfectly cold.

To make Almond Cream.

Put half a Nutmeg grated, a Bit or two of Lemon-peel, and a Blade of Mace, into a Quart of Cream, and sweeten it to your Palate; then boil them all together. In the mean time get in readiness a Quarter of a Pound of blanched Almonds that have been well beaten up with Rose and Orange-flower Water, and nine Eggs likewise well beaten, strain'd to your Almonds; which, when beat well together and rubb'd through a coarse Sieve, must be mingled with your Cream. Then pour all your Ingredients into

a Sauce-a Saucepan, set them over the Fire, and give them a gentle Boil, stirring them all the Time one Way only. When it is enough, take it off, and pour it into your Cups or Basons, but do not serve it up to Table till it is perfectly cold.

To make Ratifia Cream.

Boil six large Laurel-Leaves in a Quart of the sweetest and thickest Cream you can get, but throw the Leaves away as soon as they have been boiled long enough. In the mean Time, beat up the Yolks only of five or six Eggs with a small Quantity of cold Cream, and as much double-refined Sugar as will be agreeable. When you have thickened your Cream with your Eggs, set the Whole once more over the Fire, but take care that it does not boil, and keep stirring it all the Time one Way only. Whilst it is hot, pour it into your China Basons, and as soon as it is perfectly cold, it is fit for Use.

To make whipt Cream.

Beat up the Whites only of eight Eggs in half a Pint of Sack, and put to them a Quart of the sweetest Cream you can get; when you have stirred them all up together, add as much double-refined Sugar as will suit best with your Palate. If you like it perfumed, you may steep a little Musk or Ambergrease tied up in a Rag in your Cream. Have a Whisk in readiness, with some Lemon-peel tied up in the Middle of it, and whip your Cream up with it. Take off the Froth with a Spoon, and put it into your Glasses or Basons. *N. B.* If you design to send up any fine Tarts to Table, this whipt Cream is very proper to be laid over them.

To make whipt Syllabubs.

Grate the Peel of several Lemons into a Quart of the thickest and best Cream you can get, add thereto half a Pint of Sack, the Juice of two *Seville* Oranges, and half a Pound of the best Loaf-sugar; pour your Ingredients into a broad Pan or a deep Dish, and whisk them very well

well together; have in readiness by you some Red Wine or Sack, and put what Quantity you think convenient into your little Glasses; then as the Froth rises from your whipping the other Ingredients, take it off with a Spoon, and put it gradually into your Glasses till they are as full as they can well hold. Take notice, These Syllabubs will not keep long; therefore make but little more than what you propose shall be eaten in a few Days. It is customary with some People to make use of Cyder sweetened instead of Wine; but, in short, any Wine you like best, and sweetened to your Palate, is proper for the Purpose. Others, again, make use of Orange and Lemon Whey, made after the following Manner: Take about a Quarter of a Pint of Milk, and squeeze the Juice of an Orange or Lemon into it; as soon as your Curd is grown hard, clear the Whey from it, and sweeten it to your Taste. As to your colouring of it, you may make use either of the Juice of Saffron, Cochineal, or Spinage, according as your Inclination directs you.

To make a fine Syllabub from the Cow.

Sweeten a Quart of Cyder, or what Wine you please, with double-refined Sugar to your Palate, and grate a Nutmeg into it; then milk the Cow into your Liquor. When you have thus added what Quantity of that warm Milk you think proper, pour a Pint or more (in Proportion to the Quantity of Syllabub you make) of the sweetest Cream you can get all over it. This Syllabub may be made at home, without going to the Cow, if you think proper. You must take care, however, to have your Milk as new as you can; and, when you have set it over the Fire till it is Blood-warm, pour it out of a Tea-pot, or any other Thing of the like Nature; and, by holding your Hand very high, it will raise as good a Froth as if milk'd from the Cow.

To make everlasting Syllabubs.

To five Pints of the thickest and best Cream you can procure, add half a Pint of *Rhenish*, the same Quantity of Sack, and the Juice of two or three *Seville* Oranges, according as they are in Bigness; sweeten these Ingredients with at least a Pound of double-refined Sugar, that has been pounded to Powder and well sifted; whisk all well together with a Spoonful of Rose or Orange Water, for about half an Hour, without Intermission; then take off the Froth, and fill your Glasses with it. These Syllabubs will keep a Week or a Fortnight, and are better the Day after they are made, than to be used immediately. The best Method, however, of whipping any Syllabubs is to have ready by you a large Chocolate-Mill, which should be reserved for that particular Purpose, and a large deep Bowl to perform the Operation in: Your Froth will by that means be not only sooner raised, but will stand much stronger. Of the Thin that is left at the Bottom, you may make, if you think proper, a very fine Flummery. When you are so inclined, you must have in readiness by you a small Quantity of Calf's-Foot Jelly both boil'd and clarified. As soon as it is cold, take the Fat off, and clear it with the Whites of Eggs, and run it through a Flannel Bag; then mix it with what you reserved from your Syllabubs. When you have sweetened it with double-refined Sugar to your Taste, give it a Boil; then pour it into large China Cups or Basons. Turn it out when it is quite cold, and your Flummery is made.

To make Quince Cream.

Take Quinces when they are full ripe, cut them in Quarters, scald them till they are soft, pare them, and mash the clear Part of them and the Pulp, and put it thro' a Sieve; take an equal Weight of Quince and double-refin'd Sugar beaten and sifted, and the Whites of Eggs beat till it is as white as Snow, then put it into Dishes. You may do Apple Cream the same Way.

To make Cream of any preferv'd Fruit.

Take half a Pound of Pulp of any preferv'd Fruit, put it in a large Pan, put to it the Whites of two or three Eggs, beat them well together for an Hour, then with a Spoon take it off, and lay it heap'd up high on the Dish and Salver without Cream, to put in the middle Bason. Rafpberries will not do this Way.

To make Flummery.

Put what Quantity of Oatmeal you think convenient into a Pan that is both broad and deep, and cover it with Water, and after you have stirred it for some considerable Time, let it stand for twelve Hours, then clear off your first Water, and add fresh to your Oatmeal, and repeat it thus once in twelve Hours; then strain your Oatmeal through a coarse Sieve into a Saucepan, and set it over the Fire: Take care to keep stirring it with a Stick all the Time till it boils to a Confistence; then pour it into Dishes: As soon as it is cold, turn it into Plates, and add to it what Wine, Beer, Milk, or Cyder you think proper, and sweeten the whole to your Palate with double-refined Sugar. Take Notice, a great deal of Water must be put at first to your Oatmeal; when you pour off your last Water, you must pour no more fresh Water on than will just be sufficient to strain your Oatmeal off. Some People will let their Oatmeal stand in Water eight and forty Hours, and others for three Days succeffively, only observing to shift their Waters every twelve Hours; but that is just as Fancy directs, and as the Persons that partake of it love it either sweet or tart. Groats, however, that have been once cut, do better than Oatmeal. Every Time you add fresh Water, take care to stir it well together as you did at first.

Instructions *for making divers Sorts of Jellies.*

To make Hartshorn Jelly.

PUT Half a Pound of Hartshorn into three Quarts of Water, and boil it till it comes to a Jelly over a slow Fire, strain it before it grows cold; then put it into a Saucepan that is very well tinn'd, and add to it about a Pint of *Rhenish* Wine, and a Quarter of a Pound of double refined Sugar; when you have beat up the Whites of half a Dozen Eggs into a Froth, stir all the Ingredients well together that the Whites may be well mixed with your Jelly. When it has boiled for a few Minutes, add to it the Juice of three or four Lemons; and then give another Boil for about two Minutes. As soon as you find it very well curdled, and very white, have in Readiness your Jelly-bag, laid over a China Dish; pour your Jelly into it and back again till it is as clear as Rock Water: Thus duly prepared, fill your Glasses with a clean Spoon. Have ready for the Purpose the Rind of Lemons pared as thin as is possible, and as soon as you have half filled your Glasses throw your Peel into your Dish or Bason, over which your Bag is laid, and by that Time all your Jelly is run out, it will appear of a fine Amber Colour. As there is no certain Rule to be prescribed for putting in your Ingredients, you put what Quantity of Lemon Juice and Sugar is most agreeable to your Taste; but in the Opinion of most People they are good for very little unless they are very sweet.

To make Calves Feet Jelly.

Put two Calves Feet into a Saucepan with a Gallon of Water in it, let it boil over a gentle Fire till your Liquor is reduced to one Fourth of its Quantity, and then strain it; when it has stood till it is cold, skim off all the Fat you can that lies on the Surface. When you take up your Jelly, if you find any Sediments at the Bottom, make no Use of them; but put your clear Jelly into a Saucepan, and add to it about a Pint of Mountain Wine, half a Pound of double-refined Sugar, and the Juice of four large Lemons. Have in Readiness the Whites of about half a Dozen Eggs, or more, if you think proper, that have been well worked up with a Whisk, add them to the rest of your Ingredients in your Saucepan, and keep stirring them all well together over the Fire till they boil; in a few Minutes it will be enough. Have in Readiness a large Flannel Bag, and pour your Liquor in directly; and as it will soon run through pour it in again, till you find it run perfectly clear; then take a large China Bowl, with the Peels of your Lemons cut as thin as possibly may be, and let your Jelly run into that Bowl; for the Peels will not only give a fine Amber Colour, but a Flavour likewise. Fill your Glasses with a clean Silver Spoon.

To make Currant Jelly.

When you have stripp'd your Currants from their Stalks, throw them into a Stone Jar, and when you have stopped the Mouth of it as close as possible, set it into a Kettle of boiling Water that rises to half way of the Jar; when it has stood over the Fire for half an Hour take it off, and strain off all the Juice you find in it through a Hair-sieve. Put a Pound of double-refined Sugar to a Pint of your Juice, and then set your Ingredients over a quick clear Fire, in a Bell-Metal Skillet, and keep stirring them till all your Sugar is well dissolved; then, as you will find a Scum arises, take it very carefully and cleanly off; when your Jelly is sufficiently fine, pour it into Gallipots; when it is cold have some white Paper in Readiness cut to the exact Size of the Mouth of your Pots, then dip those Papers into a small Quantity of Brandy, and lay your Jelly upon them; then cover the Mouths close with white Paper that has Holes pricked through it. You may put some of your Jelly into Glasses if you think proper, but take Care to paper them as you do your Pots, and to keep them in a Place that is perfectly dry, that no Damp may come to them.

To make Raspberry Jelly.

To one Pint of your Currant Jelly put a Quart of Raspberries, and mash them well together; then set them over a gentle Fire in a clean Saucepan, and keep them stirring till you find them boil. About half a Dozen Minutes afterwards they will be enough; pour your Ingredients into Gallipots or Glasses, and paper them as you would your Currants. They will keep good, and have the full Flavour of the Raspberries, for two or three Years.

INSTRUCTIONS *for* Pickling.
To make the Pickle for Elder Buds.

TAKE a little Alegar or White-Wine Vinegar, and put to it two or three Blades of Mace, with a little whole Pepper and *Jamaica* Pepper, a few Bay Leaves and Salt, then put it to your Buds, and scald them two or three Times, then they are fit for Use.

To pickle Gerkins.

Take Gerkins of the finest Growth, pick them clean, put them in a strong Salt and Water, let them lie for a Week or ten Days, till they are thoroughly yellow; then scald them once a Day in the same Salt and Water they lie in, and let them lie till they are green, then set them in the Corner End, close covered.

To pickle Cucumbers.

Take a little Alegar, (the Quantity must be equal to the Quantity of your Cucumbers, and so must your Seasoning) a little Pepper, a little *Jamaica* and long Pepper, two or three Shalots, a little Horse-radish scraped or sliced, a little Salt, and a Bit of Alum; boil them all together, and scald your Cucumbers two or three Times with your Pickle, so tie them up for Use.

To make Mango of Cucumbers or small Melons.

Gather Cucumbers when they are green, cut a Bit off the End, and take out all the Meat, lay them in Salt and Water,

Water, let them lie for a Week or ten Days, till they are yellow, then ſcald them in the ſame Salt and Water they lay in whilſt green, drain from them the Water, Take a little Muſtard Seed, a little Horſe-radiſh, ſome ſcraped and ſome ſhred fine, a Handful of Shalots, a Clove or two of Garlick if you like the Taſte, and a little ſhred Mace; take ſix or eight Cucumbers ſhred fine, mix them amongſt the reſt of the Ingredients, then fill your Melons or Cucumbers with the Meat, and put in the Bits at the Ends, tie them on with a String, ſo take as much Alegar or White-Wine Vinegar as will well cover them, and put into it a little *Jamaica* and whole Pepper, a little Horſe-radiſh, and a Handful or two of Muſtard-ſeed, then boil it and pour it upon your Mango; let it ſtand in the Corner's End two or three Days, ſcald them once a Day, and then tie them up for Uſe.

To pickle Red Cabbage.

Take a Red Cabbage, chuſe it a purple Red, for the light Red never proves a good Colour; ſo take your Cabbage, and ſhred it in thin Slices, ſeaſon it with Pepper and Salt very well, let it lie all Night upon a broad Tin, or Dripping-pan; take a little Alegar, put to it a little *Jamaica* Pepper, and two or three Races of Ginger; boil them together, and when it is cold, pour it upon your Cabbage, and in two or three Days Time it will be fit for Uſe. You may throw a little Colly-flower amongſt it, and it will turn red.

To pickle Walnuts black.

Lay ſuch Nuts as are at their full Growth, but not hard, in Salt and Water for two Days, and then ſhift them into freſh Water; and there let them lie for two Days longer, and after you have ſhifted them once more, and they have laid in that Water three Days longer, then depoſit them into a Pot or Jar in which you propoſe to pickle them. Put a large Onion ſtuck with Cloves into your Jar, when it is half full. To a Hundred of your Nuts you muſt throw in half an Ounce of black Pepper, the same Quantity of All-Spice, half a dozen Bay-Leaves, a Stick of Horse-radish, a Quarter of an Ounce of Mace, and a Pint of Mustard-seed; then fill your Pot, and have some Vinegar ready boiled at hand to pour over your Nuts. Cover them with a Plate, and let them stand till they are quite cold; then tie them down with a Bladder and a Piece of Leather, and in three Months, or less, they will be fit for Use. If you have any remaining the next Year, boil your Vinegar up again, and take the Scum off as it rises. As soon as it is cold, pour it over your Nuts. You may add to it what fresh Vinegar you think proper.

To pickle Walnuts black.

Take Walnuts when they are at full Growth, and you can thrust a Pin through them, the largest Sort you can get; pare them, and cut a Bit off one End till you see the White; so you must pare off all the Green, (if you cut through the White to the Kernel, they will be spotted) and put them in Water as you pare them; you must boil them in Salt and Water, as you do Mushrooms, and they will take no more boiling than Mushrooms. When they are boiled, lay them on a dry Cloth to drain, out of the Water; then put them into a Pot, and put to them as much distilled Vinegar as will cover them; let them lie two or three Days, then take a little more Vinegar, put to it a few Blades of Mace, a little white Pepper and Salt, and boil them together. When it is cold, take your Walnuts out of the other Pickle and put into that, let them lie two or three Days, pour it from them, give it another Boil, and skim it; when it is cold, put it to your Walnuts again; put them into a Bottle, and put over them a little sweet Oil; cork them up, and set them in a cool Place. If your Vinegar be good, they will keep as long as Mushrooms.

To pickle Mushrooms.

Take Mushrooms when fresh gather'd, sort the large ones from the Buttons, cut off the Stalks, wash them in

Water with a Flannel, have a Pan of Water ready on the Fire to boil them in, for the less they lie in the Water the better; let them have two or three Boils over the Fire, then put them into a Sieve, and when you have drained the Water from them, put them into a Pot, throw over them a Handful of Salt, stop them up close with a Cloth, and let them stand two or three Hours on the hot Hearth, or the Range-End, giving your Pot a Shake now and then; then drain the Pickle from them, and lay them in a Cloth for an Hour or two, so put them into as much distilled Vinegar as will cover them; let them lie a Week or ten Days, then take them out, and put them in dry Bottles; put to them a little white Pepper, Salt, and Ginger sliced, fill them up with distilled Vinegar, put over them a little sweet Oil, and cork them up close. If your Vinegar be good, they will keep two or three Years: I know it by Experience. You must be sure not to fill your Bottles above three Parts full; if you do, they will not keep.

To pickle Collflower white.

Take the whitest Colliflower you can get, break it in Pieces the Bigness of a Mushroom, take as much distilled Vinegar as will cover it, and put to it a little white Pepper, two or three Blades of Mace, and a little Salt; then boil it, and pour it on your Colliflower three times; let it be cold, then put it into your Glasses or Pots, and wet a Bladder to tie over it to keep out the Air.

To make Catchup.

Take large Mushrooms when they are fresh gathered, cut off the dirty Ends, break them small in your Hands, put them in a Stone Bowl, with a Handful or two of Salt, and let them stand all Night. If you do not get Mushrooms enough at once, with a little Salt they will keep a Day or two till you can get more; so put them in a Stew-pot, and set them in an Oven with Houshold-Bread; when they are enough, strain from them the Liquor,

quor, and let it ſtand to ſettle; then boil it with a little Mace, *Jamaica* and whole black Pepper, two or three Shalots; boil it over a ſlow Fire for an Hour; when it is boil'd let it ſtand to ſettle, and when it is cold bottle it; if you boil it well, it will keep a Year or two. You muſt put in Spices according to the Quantity of your Catchup; you muſt not waſh them, nor put to them any Water.

To pickle Elder Buds.

Take Elder Buds when they are the Bigneſs of ſmall Walnuts, lay them in a ſtrong Salt and Water for ten Days, then ſcald them in freſh Water, and put in a Lump of Alum; let them ſtand in the Corner-End cloſe cover'd up, and ſcalded once a Day till green. You may do Radiſh Pods or Brown Buds the ſame Way.

See how to make the *Pickle*, p. 107.

To pickle French Beans.

Obſerve the ſame Method here as is before preſcribed for the pickling of your Gerkins.

To pickle Onions.

Take what Quantity of Onions you think proper, that are ſufficiently dry, and not bigger than a common Walnut; but moſt chuſe ſuch as are ſmaller. Take nothing off from them but their outward Coat; then boil them till they are tender, in one Water only; drain them thro' a Cullender, and let them lie till they are cold; after that ſtrip off their outward Skin till they be perfectly white, and then dry them with a fine ſoft Linen Cloth. In the next place, put them into wide-mouth'd Bottles fit for the Purpoſe, and throw into each Bottle half a dozen Bay-Leaves. If your Bottle holds a Quart of Onions, you muſt put to them two large Races of Ginger ſliced, and a Quarter of an Ounce of Mace; then boil two Ounces of Bay-Salt in one of Vinegar, and in proportion, be the Quantity more or leſs. As the Skin riſes, take it off, and then pour it into your Glaſſes. Cover the Mouths of your

Bottles with a Bladder that has been dipp'd in Vinegar, and tie it down. Obſerve, As you find the Pickle waſtes, you muſt fill up your Bottles with cold Vinegar.

To pickle Pigeons.

Take your Pigeons and boil them; you muſt begin to bone them at the Neck, and turn the Skin downwards. When they are boned, ſeaſon them with Pepper, Salt, and Nutmeg; ſew up both Ends, and boil them in Water and White-wine Vinegar, with a few Bay-Leaves, and a little whole Pepper and Salt; when they are enough, take them out of the Pickle, and boil it down with a little more Salt; when it is cold, put in the Pigeons, and keep them for Uſe.

To pickle Barberries.

Take Barberries when full ripe, put them into a Pot, boil a ſtrong Salt and Water, then pour it on them boiling hot.

To pickle Potatoe Crabs.

Gather your Crabs when they are young, and about the Bigneſs of a large Cherry; lay them in a ſtrong Salt and Water, as you do other Pickles; let them ſtand for a Week or ten Days, then ſcald them in the ſame Water they lay in twice a Day till green; make the ſame Pickle for them as you do for Cucumbers; be ſure you ſcald them twice or thrice in the Pickle, and they will keep the better.

To pickle large Buttons.

Take your Buttons, clean them, and cut them in three or four Pieces, put them into a large Saucepan to ſtew in their own Liquor; put to them a little *Jamaica* and whole Pepper, a Blade or two of Mace, and a little Salt; cover it up, let it ſtew over a ſlow Fire till you think they are enough, then ſtrain from them their Liquor, and put to it a little White-wine Vinegar, or Alegar, which you pleaſe, give it a Boil together, and when it is cold put it to your Muſhrooms, and keep them for Uſe. You may pickle Flaps the ſame Way.

To pickle Sprats for Anchovies.

Take an Anchovy Barrel, or a deep glazed Pot, put a few Bay Leaves at the Bottom, a Layer of Bay Salt, and some Saltpetre mixed together; than a Layer of Sprats crouded close, the Bay Leaves and the same Salt and Sprats, and so till your Barrel or Pot be full; then put in the Head of your Barrel close, and once a Week turn the other End upwards: In three Months they will be fit to eat raw as Anchovies, but they will not dissolve.

To pickle Herrings.

Scale and clean your Herrings, take out the Melts and Roes, and skewer them round, season them with a little Pepper and Salt, put them in a deep Pot, cover them with Ale Vinegar, put to them a little whole Jamaica Pepper, and two or three Bay Leaves; bake them and keep them for Use.

To pickle Sellery.

Pick Sellery two Inches in Length, set them off and let them cool; put your Pickle in cold. The Pickle for Cabbage will do this.

To pickle Turnip Tops.

Cut off the withered Leaves or Branches from your Turnip Tops, and make some Water boil, then put in your Tops, and boil them very tender, let them be cold, and put them into a Pickle of White-Wine Vinegar and Salt.

To pickle Cowslips or any other Flowers.

Take Cowslips or any other Sort of Flowers, put them into a Pot, with their Weight in Sugar, and put a Pint of Vinegar to each Pound of Sugar.

To pickle Purslain.

Take the thickest Stalks of Purslain, lay them in Salt and Water six Weeks, then take them out, put them into boiling Water, and cover them well; let them hang over a slow Fire till they are very green; when they are cold put them into a Pot, and cover them well with Beer Vinegar, and keep them cover'd close.

To pickle Nasturtium Buds.

Gather your little Buds quickly after the Blossoms are off, put them in cold Water and Salt three Days, shifting them once a Day; then make a Pickle for them (but don't boil them at all) of some White-Wine, and some White-Wine Vinegar, Shalot, Horse-radish, whole Pepper, and Salt, and a Blade or two of Mace; then put in your Seeds, and stop them close up. They are to be eaten as Capers.

To dry Pears or Pippins without Sugar.

Take Pears or Apples, and wipe them clean, take a Bodkin, and run it in at the Head, and out at the Stalk, put them in a flat earthen Pot and bake them, but not too much; you must put a Quart of strong new Ale to half a Peck of Pears, tie white Papers over the Pots that they are baked in, let them stand till cold, then drain them, squeeze the Pears flat, and the Apples the Eye to the Stalk, and lay them on Sieves with wide Holes to dry, either in a Stove or an Oven.

To preserve Mulberries whole.

Set some Mulberries over the Fire in a Skillet or Preserving-pan, draw from them a Pint of Juice when it is strained; then take three Pounds of Sugar, beaten very fine, wet the Sugar with a Pint of Juice, boil up your Sugar, and skim it, put in two Pounds of ripe Mulberries, and let them stand in the Syrup till they are thoroughly warm, then set them on the Fire, and let them boil very gently; do them but half enough, so put them by in the Syrup till next Day, then boil them gently again; when the Syrup is pretty thick, and will stand in round Drops when it is cold, they are enough, so put all in a Gally-pot for Use.

To preserve large white Plums

To a Pound of white Plums take three Quarters of a Pound of double-refin'd Sugar in Lumps, dip it in Water, boil and skim it very well, slit your Plums down the Seam;

Seam, and put them into the Syrup with the Slit downwards; let them stew over the Fire a Quarter of an Hour, skim them very well, then take them off, and when cold cover them up; turn them in the Syrup two or three Times a Day for four or five Days, then put them into Pots, and keep them for Use.

To preserve red Gooseberries.

Take a Pound of Six-penny Sugar and a little Juice of Currants, put in a Pound and a Half of red Gooseberries, and let them boil quick a Quarter of an Hour; but if they are for Jam, they must boil better than half an Hour. They are very proper for Tarts, or to eat as Sweet-Meats.

To keep Raspberries for Tarts all the Year.

Take Raspberries when they are full ripe, and pick them from the Stalk, put them into dry Bottles, cork them up very close, and keep them for Use. You may do Cranberries the same Way.

To preserve Fruit green all the Year.

Gather your Fruit when they are three Parts ripe, on a very dry Day, when the Sun shines on them, then take earthen Pots and put them in, cover the Pots with Cork, or bung them that no Air get to them, dig a Place in the Earth a Yard deep, set the Pots therein, and cover them for Use. When you take any out, cover them up again as at first.

To pickle Currants.

Take Currants either red or white before they are thoroughly ripe; you must not take them off the Stalk; make a Pickle of Salt and Water and a little Vinegar, so keep them for Use. These are proper for Garnishing.

The *British* VINTNER:

Containing DIRECTIONS *for making all Sorts of* WINES.

To make Elder Wine.

TAKE twenty Pounds of *Malaga* Raisins, pick and chop them, then put them into a Tub, with twenty Quarts of Water, let the Water be boiled, and stand till it be cold again, before you put in your Raisins; let them remain together ten Days, stirring it twice a Day; then strain the Liquor very well from the Raisins, through a Canvas-strainer or Hair-sieve; add to it six Quarts of Elder Juice, five Pounds of Loaf-sugar, and a little Juice of Sloes, to make it acid, just as you please; put it into a Vessel, and let it stand in a pretty warm Place three Months, then bottle it; the Vessel must be stopped till it has done working. If your Raisins are very good, you may leave out the Sugar.

To make Gooseberry Wine.

Pick, clean, and beat your Gooseberries in a Marble Mortar or wooden Bowl, measure them in Quarts heaped up, add two Quarts of Spring Water, and let them stand all Night, or twelve Hours; then rub or press out the Husks very well, strain them through a wide Strainer, and to every Gallon put three Pounds of Sugar, and a Gill of Brandy; then put all into a sweet Vessel, not very full, and keep it very close for four Months, then decant it off till it comes clear, pour out the Grounds and wash the Vessel clean, with a little of the Wine; add to every Gallon a Pound more Sugar, let it stand a Month in the Vessel again, drop the Grounds through a Flannel Bag, and put it to the other Vessel; the Tap-hole must not be
too

too near the Bottom of the Cask, for fear of letting out the Grounds.

The same Receipt will serve for Currant Wine the same Way. Let them be red Currants.

To make Balm-Wine.

Take a Peck of Balm-leaves, put them into a Tub or large Pot, heat four Gallons of Water scalding hot ready to boil, then pour it upon the Leaves; so let it stand all Night, then strain them through a Hair-sieve; put to every Gallon of Water two Pounds of fine Sugar, and stir it very well; take the Whites of four or five Eggs, beat them very well, put them into a Pan, and whisk it very well before it be too hot; when the Skim begins to rise, take it off, and keep it skimming all the while it is boiling; let it boil three Quarters of an Hour, then put it into the Tub; when it is cold put a little new Yeast upon it, and beat it every two Hours, that it may head the better; so work it up for two Days, then put it into a sweet Roundlet, bung it up close, and when it is fine bottle it.

To make Raisin Wine.

Take ten Gallons of Water, and fifty Pounds of *Malaga* Raisins, pick out the large Stalks, and boil them in your Water; when your Water is boiled, put it into a Tub; take the Raisins, and chop them very small; when your Water is blood-warm, put in your Raisins, and rub them very well with your Hand; when you put them into the Water, let them work for ten Days, stirring them twice a Day; then strain out the Raisins in a Hair-sieve, and put them into a clean hardened Bag, and squeeze it in the Press, to take out the Liquor, so put it into your Barrel; do not let it be too full, bung it up close, and let it stand till it is fine; when you tap your Wine, you must not tap it too near the Bottom, for fear of the Grounds; when it is drawn off, take the Grounds out of the Barrel, and wash it out with a little of your Wine; then put your Wine into the Barrel again, draw your Grounds through a Flana Flannel Bag, and put them into the Barrel to the reſt; add to it two Pounds of Loaf-ſugar, then bung it up, and let it ſtand a Week or ten Days; if it be very ſweet to your Taſte, let it ſtand ſome Time longer, and bottle it.

To make Birch Wine.

Take your Birch-Water, and boil it, clear it with Whites of Eggs; to every Gallon of Water take two Pounds and a Half of fine Sugar, boil it three Quarters of an Hour, and when it is almoſt cold, put in a little Yeaſt, work it two or three Days, then put it into the Barrel, and to every five Gallons put in a Quart of Brandy, and half a Pound of ſtoned Raiſins; before you put up your Wine, burn a Brimſtone-Match in the Barrel.

To make white Currant Wine.

Take the largeſt white Currants you can get, ſtrip and break them in your Hand, till you break all the Berries; to every Quart of Pulp take a Quart of Water, let the Water be boiled, and cold again; mix them well together, let them ſtand all Night in your Tub, then ſtrain them through a Hair-ſieve, and to every Gallon put two Pounds and a Half of Six-penny Sugar; when your Sugar is diſſolved, put it into your Barrel, diſſolve a little Iſinglaſs, whiſk it with Whites of Eggs, and put it in: To every four Gallons put in a Quart of Mountain Wine, ſo bung up the Barrel; when it is fine, draw it off, and take off the Grounds, (but do not tap the Barrel too low at the Bottom) waſh out the Barrel with a little of your Wine, and drop the Grounds through a Bag; then put it to the reſt of your Wine, and put it all into your Barrel again; to every Gallon add half a Pound more of Sugar, and let it ſtand another Week or two; if it be too ſweet, let it ſtand a little longer, then bottle it off and it will keep two or three Years.

To make Cowſlip Wine.

Take ten Gallons of Water, when it is almoſt boiling, add to it twenty-one Pounds of fine Powder-fugar, let it boil half an Hour, and fkim it very clean; when it is boiled put it in a Tub, let it ftand till you think it be cold enough to fet on the Yeaft; take a Porringer of new Yeaft off the Vat, and put to it a few Cowflips; when you put on the Yeaft, put in a few every Time it is ftirr'd, till all the Cowflips be in, which muft be fix Pecks, and let it work three or four Days; add to it fix Lemons, cut off the Peel, and the Infides put into your Barrel, then add to it a Pint of Brandy; when you think it has done working, clofe up your Veffel, let it ftand a Month, and then bottle it; you may let your Cowflips lie a Week or ten Days to dry before you take your Wine, for it makes it much finer; you may put in a Pint of White-Wine that is good, inftead of the Brandy.

To make Orange Wine.

Take fix Gallons of Water, and fifteen Pounds of Powder-fugar, the Whites of fix Eggs well beaten, boil them three Quarters of an Hour, and fkim them while any Skim will rife; when it is cold enough for working, put to it fix Ounces of the Syrup of Citron or Lemons, and fix Spoonfuls of Yeaft, beat the Syrup and Yeaft well together, and put in the Peel and Juice of fifty Oranges, work it two Days and a Night; then tun it up into a Barrel, fo bottle it at three or four Months old.

To make Orange Brandy.

Take a Quart of Brandy, the Peels of eight Oranges pared thin, fteep them in Brandy forty-eight Hours, in a clofe Pitcher; then take three Pints of Water, put into it three Quarters of a Pound of Loaf Sugar, boil it till Half be confumed, and let it ftand till it be cold, then mix it with the Brandy.

To make Punch.

Take a Quart or two of Sherbet before you put in your Brandy, and the Whites of four or five Eggs, beat them very well, and fet it over the Fire, let it have a Boil, then

put

it into a Jelly-Bag, so mix the rest of your Acid and Brandy together, (the Quantity you design to make) heat it and run it all through your Jelly-Bag, change it in the running off till it looks fine; let the Peel of one or two Lemons lie in the Bag; you may make it the Day before you use it, and bottle it.

To make Orange Ale.

Take forty *Seville* Oranges, pare and cut them in Slices, the best coloured *Seville* you can get, put them all with the Juice and Seeds into Half an Hogshead of Ale; when it is tunned up and working, put in the Oranges, and at the same Time a Pound and a Half of Raisins of the Sun stoned; when it is done working, close up the Bung, and it will be ready to drink in a Month.

Cyprus *Wine imitated.*

Put nine Quarts of the Juice of white Elder-Berries which has been pressed gently from the Berries with the Hand, and pressed through a Sieve without bruising the Kernels of the Berries, to nine Gallons of Water; add to every Gallon of Liquor three Pounds of *Lisbon* Sugar, and to the whole Quantity put an Ounce and a Half of Ginger sliced, and three Quarters of an Ounce of Cloves, then boil this near an Hour, taking off the Scum as it rises, and pour the whole to cool in an open Tub, and work it with Ale Yeast spread upon a Toast of white Bread three Days, and then turn it into a Vessel that will just hold it, adding about a Pound and a Half of Raisins of the Sun split, to lie in the Liquor till you draw it off, which should not be till the Wine is fine, which you will find in *January*. This is so much like the fine rich Wine brought from *Cyprus*, in its Colour and Flavour, that it has deceived the very best of Judges.

To make Hungary Water.

Put half a Peck of Rosemary Flowers to a Gallon of strong Spirits. Infuse them in the Spirits for a Fortnight, and then distil them.

To make Mead.

Put sixty Quarts of Water to five Quarts of Honey, eighteen Races of sliced Ginger, and one Handful of Rosemary, let them boil three Hours, and be scum'd perpetually; when cold, put your Yeast to it, and it will be fit to bottle in about eight or ten Days.

Directions for BREWING.

The Method of Brewing Ale or Beer.

PUT sixteen Gallons of Water into your Copper, strew over it as much Bran as will cover it, make it scalding hot, then put a third Part of it into the Mashing-Tub, where let it stand till the Steam is so far spent that you can see your Face in your Liquor; then put to it a Bushel of Malt, and stir it very well into the Liquor. In the mean while make the rest of the Water left in the Copper boil; then either damp or put out the Fire under the Copper, that the Liquor may be allayed in its Heat; and then put it into the Mashing-Tub, and stir it all well together. If you suspect any ill Taint in the Malt, you may throw in a Shovel or two of hot Coals to take it off. While this Liquor stands upon the Malt in the Mashing-Tub, heat sixteen Gallons more of Liquor, and having drawn off your first Wort, put Part of it upon the Grains, and put in three Pecks more of fresh Malt; then put the first Wort into the Copper again, make it scalding hot, and put Part of it into a second Mashing-Tub, and when the Steam is over, stir in it three Pecks more of fresh Malt, then put in the rest of the Water, and stir it well, letting it stand two Hours; then heat another sixteen Gallons of Water, and after that which was put into the first Mash-Tub has stood two Hours, draw it off, and also the Wort which is in the second Mashing-Tub, and put the Grains out of the second Mashing-Tub into the first; and put into it the Liquor in the Copper, and let it stand an Hour and a half. If you would have Beer, boil the first Wort with half a Pound of Hops for two Hours, or till it looks curdled, and for Ale, boil the second Wort with three Ounces of Hops for an Hour and a half; and boil the Hops of both Worts for an Hour and a half in the other Liquor for Table-Beer.

To recover Beer that is flat or dead.

Take four Gallons out of a Hogshead, and boil it with five Pounds of Honey, scum it, let it be cooled, and put it to the rest; stop it up close, and it will make it pleasant, quick, and strong.

To make stale Beer drink new.

Stamp the Herb Horehound, strain the Juice, and put a Spoonful of it to a Quart or three Pints of Beer; cover it, let it stand two Hours, and then drink it.

To put a stop to Beer upon the Fret.

Pour a Quart of Black Cherry Brandy into a Hogshead of Beer, and stop it up close.

To make Beer, Ale, or any other Malt Liquors fine.

Put half an Ounce of unslacked Lime into a Pint of Water, and having mixed them well together, let them stand three Hours, and by that Time the Lime will have settled to the Bottom; pour off the clear Water from the Lime, and put it into Ale or Beer, first mixing with it half an Ounce of Isinglass cut small and boiled; and in five Hours Time, or less, the Beer in the Barrel will be settled and clear.

A Method of brewing Ale, *or* October Beer, *from* Nottingham.

Supposing the Copper to hold 24 Gallons, and the Mashing-Tub large enough to hold four Bushels or more of Malt, the first full Copper of boiling Water is put into the Mashing-Tub, and having laid on the Malt for a

Quarter of an Hour till the Steam is so far spent that one can see his Face in it, or as soon as the hot Water is put in; put into it a Pailful or two of cold Water, which at once brings it into Temper; then three Bushels of Malt are poured leisurely into it, being stirred or mashed all the while it is putting in; but as little as can be, or no more than will just keep the Malt from clotting or balling: This being done, one Bushel of dry Malt is put on the Top to keep in the Vapour or Spirit, then cover it up and let it stand for two Hours, or till another Copper full of Water is boiling hot; this is laded over the Malt by three Hand-bowls full at a Time, which are to run off at the Cock or Tap by a very small Stream before more is put in; which again is returned into the Mash-Tub till it comes off exceeding fine; for if the Wort is not clear when it is put into the Copper, there are but small Hopes it will be so in the Barrel. The brewing after this leisurely Manner requires sixteen Hours to brew four Bushels of Malt. Now between the Ladings out of the Copper, cold Water is put into the Copper to be boiling hot, while the other is running off, and by this Means the Copper is kept near full, and the Cock spending till near the End of brewing either Ale or small Beer, of which no more than twenty-one Gallons are to be saved of the first Wort, which is reserved in a Tub, then four Ounces of Hops are put in, and then it is set by. For the second Wort, suppose there are twenty Gallons of Water in the Copper boiling hot, that must be all laded over in the same Manner as the former was, but no cold Water need here be mixed: When half of this is run out into the Tub, it must directly be put into the Copper, with half of the first Wort, strained through a brewing Sieve, as it lies on a small loose wooden Frame, over the Copper, to keep back those Hops which were first put in to preserve it; which is to make the first Copper twenty-one Gallons. Then, upon its beginning to boil, a Pound of Hops is put into one or two Canvas or other coarse Linen Bags, something larger

M 2   than

than will just contain the Hops, that they may have Room to swell; these boiled briskly for half an Hour, then the Hops are taken out, and the Wort is continued boiling by itself till it breaks into Particles a little ragged, and then it is enough, and may be dispersed into the cooling Vessels very thin. Then the Remainder of the first and second Wort are put together at the same Time, in the same Manner, and with the same Quantity of fresh Hops as the first was. The rest of the third or small Beer Wort will be about fifteen or twenty Gallons, more or less; this is directly mixed with cold Water to keep it free from Excise, and this is put into the Copper as the first Brewing of Ale with another four Bushels of Malt as was done before, and so on for several Days together, if necessary; but at last there may be some small Beer made, yet some make none, but make use of the Grains in feeding their Hogs.

To make Dr. Butler's Purging Ale.

Take Polypody of the Oak, and Sena, of each a Quarter of a Pound, Sarsaparilla two Ounces, Aniseeds and Carraway-seeds of each an Ounce, of Scurvy-Grass half a Bushel, Agrimony and Maiden-Hair of each a Handful; bruise all these moderately in a Mortar, and put them into a Canvas Bag, and hang them in three Gallons of Ale: Let it stand three Days, and it will be drinkable.

Ale of Health, according to the Recipe of the Viscount St. Alban's.

Take of Sarsaparilla three Ounces; Sassafras Wood and China Root, of each half a Ounce; of Mace a Quarter of an Ounce; white Saunders and Champitityon, of each an Ounce. Let the Wood be sliced as thin as can be, and all be bruised together in a Mortar: Then add *Roman* Wormwood, Hops, and Cowslip Flowers, of each two Handfuls; Sage, Rosemary, Sweet Marjoram, Balm, Mugwort, and Betony, all together four Handfuls. Boil all these together in six Gallons of Ale, till it is consumed to four; then put the Wood and Ale into six Gallons of
the

the second Wort, and boil it to four Gallons; then let all the Ale run from the Dregs, mix it together, and put it up in a Vessel.

The FAMILY PHYSICIAN.

A Receipt for a Hoarseness upon a Cold.

TAKE three Ounces of Hyssop Water, sweeten it with Sugar-Candy, and beat the Yolk of an Egg well into it.

For the Head-Ach.

Make Vinegar of Vervain as you make Vinegar of Roses, only make it of the Leaves, not of the Flower of Vervain; bathe the Head with it.

For a Corn on the Toe.

Take a black Snail and roast it well in a white wet Cloth, bruise it, and lay it hot to the Corn, and it will take it away in a very short Time.

For Warts.

Anoint your Warts with Pigeons Dung, mixed with Vinegar, and it will cure them.

For a Quartan Ague.

Rue bruised, and worn under the Feet next the Skin, is an excellent Remedy.

The following Receipts were inserted in the Carolina *Gazette,* May 9, 1750.

To the PRINTER.

SIR,

I AM commanded by the Commons-House of Assembly to send you the inclosed, which you are to print in the *Carolina* Gazette as soon as possible. It is the Negro Cæ-

sar's Cure for Poison, and likewise his Cure for the Bite of a Rattle-Snake: For discovering of which the General Assembly hath thought fit to purchase his Freedom, and grant him an Allowance of 100 l. *per Annum* during his Life.

May 9, 1750.   I am, *&c.*

JAMES IRVING.

The Negro Cæsar's *Cure for Poison.*

Take the Roots of Plantane, and wild Horehound, fresh or dry, three Ounces, boil them together in two Quarts of Water till it comes to one, and strain it: Of this Decoction let the Patient take one third Part three Mornings fasting successively, from which, if he finds any Relief, it must be continued till he is perfectly recovered On the contrary, if he finds no Alteration after the third Dose, it is a Sign the Patient has either not been poisoned at all, or that it has been with such Poison as *Cæsar*'s Antidotes will not remedy; so may leave off the Decoction.

During the Cure, the Patient must live on a spare Diet, and abstain from eating Mutton, Pork, Butter, or any other fat or oily Food.

N. B. The Plantane or Horehound will either of them cure alone, but they are most efficacious together. In the Summer you may take a Handful of the Roots and Branches of each, in place of three Ounces of the Roots of each.

For Drink during the Cure, let them take the following;

Take of the Roots of Golden Rod, six Ounces, or in Summer two large Handfuls, the Roots and Branches together, and boil them in two Quarts of Water to one Quart (to which may be added a little Horehound and Sassafras.) To this Decoction, after it is strained, add a Glass of Rum or Brandy, and sweeten it with Sugar for an ordinary Drink.

Some-

Sometimes an inward Fever attends such as are poison'd, for which he orders the following:

Take a Pint of Wood Ashes and three Pints of Water, stir it and mix them well together, let them stand all Night, and strain or decant the Lye off in the Morning, of which ten Ounces may be taken six Mornings following, warmed or cold according to the Weather. These Medicines have no sensible Operation, though sometimes they work in the Bowels and give a gentle Stool.

The Symptoms attending such as are poison'd, are as follow:

A Pain of the Breast, Difficulty of breathing, a Load at the Pit of the Stomach, an irregular Pulse, burning and violent Pains of the Viscera above and below the Navel, very restless at Night, sometimes wandering Pains over the whole Body, a Retching and Inclination to vomit, profuse Sweats (which prove always serviceable) slimy Stools, both when costive and loose, the Face of a pale yellow Colour, sometimes a Pain and Inflammation of the Throat, the Appetite is generally weak, and some cannot eat any; those who have been long poisoned are generally very feeble and weak in their Limbs, sometimes spit a great deal, the whole Skin peels, and likewise the Hair falls off.

Cæsar's Cure for the Bite of a Rattle-Snake.

Take of the Roots of Plantane or Horehound, (in the Summer Roots and Branches together) a sufficient Quantity, bruise them in a Mortar, and squeeze out the Juice, of which give, as soon as possible, one large Spoonful; if he is swelled you must force it down his Throat; this generally will cure; but if the Patient finds no Relief in an Hour after, you may give another Spoonful, which never fails. If the Roots are dried, they must be moistened with a little Water. To the Wound may be applied a Leaf of good Tobacco moistened in Rum.

Dr.

Dr. Mead's *Account of a Person bit by a Mad Dog. For further Particulars see his Essay of the Mad Dog, Page* 129. *And likewise his infallible Receipt for the Cure.*

The Wound from the Bite of a *Mad Dog* differs not at all from that made by a common Bite, and is as easily healed; and it is usually a confiderable Time before any bad Confequences appear. There are Inftances where thefe have been deferred to three, four, or fix Months; nay, fome Authors fay, to a Year and longer. *Galen* † himfelf faw one Cafe after a Year: I remember one after eleven Months; but the Attack is generally between thirty and forty Days, tho' very often fooner, fometimes in fifteen or fixteen Days, in younger Subjects.

The firft Approaches of the Diftemper generally difcover themfelves after this Manner. A Pain is felt in the Part which was wounded, which by Degrees fpreads itfelf to the neighbouring Parts; a Laffitude follows with Uneafinefs in all the Limbs. Then the Patient grows penfive and fad, with difturbed and unquiet Sleeps, Complaints of Faintnefs and Lownefs of Spirits, particularly of an Oppreffion at his Breaft. His Pulfe intermits, his Nerves tremble, he has cold Sweats, a great Naufea and Sicknefs at Stomach, and loaths Food; and tho' he has an inward Heat and Thirft, and defires to drink, yet he fwallows Meat, but efpecially Liquor, with great Difficulty. Thefe Symptoms increafe, and the next Day, from the great Uneafinefs and Pain which he finds in fwallowing, he conceives fuch an Averfion to Liquids, that at firft Sight of them he falls into *Convulfions* and Agonies, and cannot get down the leaft Drop. *This Hydrophobia* * has always been accounted the fureft Sign and Mark of this Poifon, by which it

† An eminent Phyfician of *Pergamus.*

* Occafioned by the Bite of a Mad Dog, wherein the Perfon hath a Dread of Water, neither can he bear the Sight of any Sort of Liquor, without violent Emotions, nor fwallow the leaft Drop, which renders the Perfon incurable.

is diſtinguiſhed from all other Diſeaſes; as not being obſerved, at leaſt very rarely, in any other Caſe whatſoever.

At this Time a Fever uſually appears, with a quick
and low Pulſe, without the leaſt Sleep, a hoarſe Voice,
a gathering of Froth in the Mouth, and ſpitting of it upon
the Standers by: Univerſal Convulſions, particularly
above the Throat, and in the *Muſculi erectores Penis*,
whence a Priapiſm is obſerved. During this tragical
Scene, which always proves fatal in about two Days, a
Delirium comes on, ſometimes with moſt terrible Symptoms of Rage and Fury, and Attempts of doing all poſ-
ſible Miſchief even to the moſt beloved Friends and Rela-
tions; but more commonly without any *Furor*, it is of the
melancholy Kind, and the Wretch reſigns to Death, and
prepares for it, bids thoſe about him take Care of themſelves, leſt he ſhould do them a Miſchief; and begs to
be troubled no more: And his Breath growing ſhorter and
ſhorter, he expires in convulſive Fits.

It is common to them all, that they can ill bear the
Impreſſion of Objects upon themſelves. All Feeling is
painful. The ſlighteſt Touch or rubbing of the Limbs
hurts, the leaſt Noiſe is offenſive, and the opening or
ſhutting of a Door affrights, as if the Houſe was falling;
the Eyes ſo ill bear the Light, that when the Sight of any
Thing white appears it is intolerable. In like Manner the
inner Membranes are ſo tender, that they can't ſuffer their
natural Senſation, the common Coolneſs of freſh Air is diſ-
agreeable to the Lungs, and the making of Water gives
Uneaſineſs and Pain in the urinal Paſſages. The Aſ-
pect is diſmal, either frightful with Tokens of Rage and
Fury, or lamentable with Marks of Moaning and De-
ſpair. There's no Sleep from the Beginning of the Fever
to the End.

When the Symptoms are *Maniacal*, the Strength of the
Muſcles are prodigious: Theſe acting indeed with a convulſive Force ſo great, that I have ſeen a Caſe, in which
a Man tied down in Bed with ſtrong Cords broke them
all

all at once by one Effort, and immediately died paralytic; as if all the Fibres of the Body had been over-ſtrained, and torn to Pieces by their violent Action.

At firſt the Patient has no Dread of Water, nor any Averſion to Liquors. On the contrary, he ſees them with Pleaſure; being thirſty, he deſires to drink, and then ſoon wonders what ſhould be the Reaſon that he is not able to take it. He contrives Ways to do it, by endeavouring to ſuck it through a Quill, but ſoon cries out it is impoſſible; when aſked why, he anſwers, It will not go down, it ſtrangles him, and begs to be excuſed trying any more.

The Receipt.

Let the Patient be blooded in the Arm nine or ten Ounces. Take the Herb called in Latin *Lichen Cinereus Terreſtris*, in Engliſh *Aſh-colour'd Ground Liverwort*, clean'd, dry'd, and powder'd, half an Ounce; of black Pepper powder'd two Drachms. Mix theſe well together, and divide the Powder into four Doſes, one of which muſt be taken every Morning faſting, for four Mornings ſucceſſively, in half a Pint of Cow's Milk warm. After theſe four Doſes are taken, the Patient muſt go into the cold Bath, or a cold Spring or River, every Morning faſting, for a Month: He muſt be dipt all over, but not ſtay in (with his Head) longer than half a Minute, if the Water be very cold; after this he muſt go in three Times a Week for a Fortnight longer.

N. B. The Lichen is a very common Herb, and grows generally in ſandy and barren Soils all over *England*. The right Time to gather it is in the Months of *October* and *November*.

For ſweating in the Night in a Conſumption.

Drink a Glaſs of Tent, or old *Malaga*, with a Toaſt every Morning early, and ſleep an Hour after it. This is good for conſumptive People, or ſuch as are weak in recovering after a long Sickneſs.

A good Drink for a Consumption.

Take St. *John*'s Wort, the largest Daisy Flower (called Ox-Eyes) and Scabius, of each a Handful, boil these in two Quarts of Spring Water till it be wasted to one Half; then strain and sweeten it with clarified Honey to your Palate Take a Quarter of a Pint of this in half a Pint of Milk, making the Liquor just Milk-warm, in the Morning, and at Four in the Afternoon. This Drink is highly commended upon long Experience.

For a dry husking Cough.

Drink a Pint of Spring Water as hot as you can at Night going to bed. This, though it seems but a trifling Remedy, has far outdone the Expectations of those that have tried it.

For a Cancer in the Mouth and Gums.

Mix 20 Drops of Spirit of Vitriol in half an Ounce of Honey of Roses. Keep the sore Place always moist with this Mixture, and it is a certain Cure.

To fasten the Teeth and preserve the Gums.

Take one Dram of Allum, two Drams of Bole Armoniac, and half a Dram of Myrrh, reduce them to a fine Powder, put it into a Pint of Claret in a Glass Bottle, stir it some Time, and wash the Teeth with it daily.

To close up the Gums and Teeth that are loose.

Calcine Earth-Worms, and rub the Teeth with the Powder; or dry a Calf's Liver in an Oven, reduce it to Powder, adding an equal Quantity of Honey to it, and bring the whole into the Consistence of Opiate.

To whiten the Teeth.

Dip a Bit of Cloth into some Vinegar of Squills, and rub the Teeth and Gums with it; for besides the whitening of them, it will also fasten and strengthen the Roots, and sweeten the Breath.

To help Children to breed their Teeth.

Take the Brains of a Hare that has either been boiled

or roasted, and mix the Brains with Honey and Butter, and rub the Child's Gums frequently with Sugar.

To make a Necklace for a Child.

Take 20 Corns of whole Pepper, and steep them in a Glass of the best Gin for an Hour, and then thread them on white Silk and tie them round the Child's Neck, and let it remain till they drop off, which they will do as the Child cuts its Teeth.

To give certain Ease in the Tooth-Ach

Take *French* Flies, Mithridate, and a few Drops of Vinegar, beat this to a Paste, and lay a Plaister on the Cheek-Bone or behind the Ear; it will draw a Blister, but rarely fails to cure.

For the Scurvy in the Teeth.

Heat a Piece of Steel red hot, and quench it half a score times in White-wine Vinegar, as fast as you can heat it; then add to the Quantity of half a Pint, a Quarter of an Ounce of Myrrh in Powder, and a Dram or two of Mastich in Powder: With this wash the Teeth three times a Day or oftener.

For the Scurvy.

Take Garden Scurvy-grass half a Peck, Brook-lime and Water-cresses, of each two Handfuls; Ground-ivy, Fir-tree Tops, Liver-wort, and Tamarisk, of each a Handful; Horse-radish Roots, Sassafras, and Daucus-seed, of each half an Ounce; Roots of sharp-pointed Dock 2 Ounces, and a large *Seville* Orange sliced; bruise all these gently, and put them into a Canvas Bag, which hang in three Gallons of Ale: When it is fine, drink a Draught of it in a Morning, or at any Time of the Day. This is one of the Prescriptions of Serjeant *Barnard*, and is an excellent Medicine for this Distemper; but where the Scurvy is also attended with the Dropsy, so that the Legs swell, the Juices of the Herbs, with the Juice of *Seville* Oranges, will be a more speedy and effectual Remedy to those whose Stomach can bear them.

For the Dropsy.

Mix six Ounces of Syrup of Elder Berries with three Ounces of Oil of Turpentine; incorporate them well together, and take a good Spoonful of this Mixture the first Thing in a Morning, and the last at Night, for a Fortnight. Some affirm, that the constant eating Sea Biscuit, and new Raisins of the Sun, instead of Suppers, has cured the Dropsy without Physick; especially if the Patient can refrain from drinking small Liquors.

Shortness of Breath.

Take half an Ounce of Elecampane Root, an Ounce of Powder of Liquorice, and the same Quantity of Flour of Brimstone and Powder of Anniseed, and a Quarter of a Pound of Sugar-Candy powdered; make all into a Mass, with a sufficient Quantity of Tar, of which take four Pills when you are going to Rest. This is likewise an excellent Medicine for an Asthma.

Another for the same.

Take Elecampane Root finely powdered, and Flour of Brimstone, in equal Quantities, mix them into an Electuary with clarified Honey, and take it whenever you are seized with the Cough, or find any Difficulty in breathing.

For the Gravel.

Boil half a Pint of Ale, scumming it very clean, then take it off the Fire, till you have beaten the Yolks of two new laid Eggs with a Spoonful of Honey; mix this with the Ale when it is so cool as not to curdle, and drink this for nine Mornings.

For the Cholic.

Infuse an Ounce of Hiera Picra in a Quart of double-distilled Anniseed Water, stop it very close and let it stand near the Fire for some Days, shaking the Bottle twice a Day. Take three or four Spoonfuls of this in a Fit when it is new; if it stands a Year or more less will serve.

For the Piles.

Boil a Handful of the Leaves of the Herb Mullein in a Pint of Milk, and sweeten it with an Ounce of Syrup of Violets, and drink every Night when you go to Bed for five or six Weeks, and it will certainly remove the Cause of the Distemper.

For an Asthma.

Roast four Cloves of Garlick till they are soft, then bruise out the Pulp, and put it into four Spoonfuls of Honey, two Spoonfuls of powdered Elecampane; of Anniseeds, Coriander, and Liquorice, all finely powdered and sifted, one Spoonful and a Half, of which take the Bigness of a Nutmeg Morning and Evening.

For a Looseness and Gripes.

Take one Dram of *Venice* Treacle, three Drops of the Oil of Juniper, and as many of the Oil of Cinnamon, which mix with twenty Grains of Rhubarb; make this into a Bolus, and take it at Night when you go to Bed. The next Morning when it works, drink warm Posset Drink, in which Mallows have been infused. This has effected Cures when the Case has been very dangerous.

For a Bruise.

Make a Poultice of Bran and Urine and apply it to the Bruise as hot as you can bear; if it be very bad, repeat it as it cools; and do it as soon after the Hurt as you can, to prevent its swelling, which the Air is apt to cause.

For a Fever.

At the Beginning of a Fever, or when the Party rageth, take Sheeps Lights and lay to the Soles of the Feet, and it will draw it quite out of the Head. Sometimes it causeth a Looseness, but then comfortable Things must be given.

For the Itch.

Make an Ointment with Flour of Brimstone and fresh Butter or Oil of Olive, and rub the Body with it Morning and Evening.

For the Jaundice.

Cut off the Top of a *Seville* Orange, take out the middle Core and Seeds as well as you can, without the Juice; fill the Vacancy with Saffron, and lay the Top on again; then roast it carefully without burning, and throw it into a Pint of White Wine. Drink a Quarter of a Pint of this fasting for nine Days, it exceedingly sweetens and clears the Blood.

To stop Bleedings immediately.

Dip a Piece of black Bays in the sharpest Vinegar, and lay it to the Patient's Groin; as it grows warm dip it again. It gives a sudden Check, and is the Practice in the *West Indies*, among the Blacks, who are subject to this Distemper, and often lost by the Violence of it. This doth seldom fail in Extremity.

For Convulsion Fits.

Mix simple Peony, and black Cherry Water, in equal Quantities, the Quantity of a Draught; into which, for a Child, put of Spirits of Hartshorn five Drops, for a Woman 20, and for a Man 30.

For a Looseness and Bloody Flux.

Put the Yolks of two new laid Eggs into a Glass of strong Cinnamon Water, Brandy, Rum, Rosa Solis, or any spirituous Liquor, and drink it all up; though these hot Things are not so proper to be used but in the greatest Extremity. Chewing of Rhubarb is as certain, and carries of the Cause.

For the Stone and Gravel.

Take two Drams of the Powder of Wood-Lice in an Ounce of Brandy, and a Pint of the Decoction of Chick-Pease. Divide this Quantity into Half, to be taken two Mornings together fasting.

To cure the Ague

Mix the Powder of White Hellebore Roots with right *Venice* Turpentine till it is stiff enough to spread on Leather. Lay the Plaister over the Wrist, and over the Ball of the Thumb, six Hours before the coming of the cold Fit.

Instructions for CARVING.

To unjoint a Bittern.

RAISE the Wings and Legs as a Hern, which see, and use no other Sauce but Salt.

To cut up a Bustard. See Turkey.

To unlace a Coney.

Turn the Back downward, and cut the Flaps or Apron from the Belly or Kidney; then put in your Knife between the Kidnies, and loosen the Flesh from the Bone on each Side, then turn the Belly downward, and cut the Back across between the Wings, drawing your Knife down on each Side the Back-bone, dividing the Legs and Sides from the Back: Pull not the Leg too hard, when you open the Side from the Bone, but with your Hand and Knife neatly lay open both Sides from the Scut to the Shoulder; then lay the Legs close together.

To display a Crane.

Unfold his Legs, then cut off his Wings by the Joints; after this, take up his Legs and Wings, and sauce them with Vinegar, Salt, Mustard, and powder'd Ginger.

To unbrace a Duck or Mallard.

Raise up the Pinions and Legs, but take them not off, and raise the Merry-thought from the Breast; then lace it down each Side of the Breast with your Knife. After the same Manner unbrace a Mallard.

To rear a Goose.

Take off both Legs fair, like Shoulders of Lamb; then cut off the Belly-piece round close to the End of the Breast; then lace your Goose down on both Sides of the Breast Half an Inch from the sharp Bone; then take off the Pinion on each Side, and the Flesh you first laced with your Knife, then raise it up clean from the Bone, and take it off with the Pinion from the Body; then cut up the Merry-thought; then cut from the Breast-bone another Slice of Flesh, quite through; then turn up your Carcase, and cut it asunder, the Back-bones above the Loin-bones.

To dismember a Hern.

Take off both the Legs, and lace it down the Breast on both Sides with your Knife, and open the Breast-Pinion, but take it not off; then raise up the Merry-thought, between the Breast-bone and the Top of it; then raise up the Brawn, and turn it outward on both Sides, but break it not, nor cut it off; then cut off the Wing-Pinions at the Joint next the Body, and stick in each Side the Pinion in the Place you turned the Brawn out: But cut off the sharp End of the Pinion, and take the Middle-piece, and that will just fit in the Place. You may cut up a Capon or Pheasant the same Way.

To wing a Partridge or Quail.

Raise the Legs and Wings, and sauce them with Wine, powder'd Ginger, and Salt.

To allay a Pheasant or Teal.

Do this as you do a Partridge, but use no other Sauce but Salt.

To lift a Swan.

Slit the Swan down in the Middle of the Breast, and so clean through the Back from the Neck to the Rump:

Then part it into two Halves, but do not break or tear the Flesh; then lay the two Halves in a Charger, with the two slit Sides downwards; throw Salt upon it; set it again upon the Table: Let the Sauce be Chaldron, and serve it in Saucers.

To cut up a Turkey.

Raise up the Leg fairly, and open the Joint with the Point of your Knife, but take not off the Leg; then with your Knife lace down both Sides of the Breast, and open the Breast-Pinion, but do not take it off; then raise the Merry-thought betwixt the Breast-bone, and the Top of it; then raise up the Brawn; then turn it outward upon both Sides, but break it not, nor cut it off; then cut off the Wing-Pinions at the Joint next the Body, and stick each Pinion in the Place you turned the Brawn out; but cut off the sharp End of the Pinion, and take the Middle-piece, and that will just fit the Place. You may cut up a Bustard, a Capon, or a Pheasant the same Way.

To thigh a Woodcock.

Raise the Wings and Legs as you do a Hern, only lay the Head open for the Brains; and as you thigh a Hern, so you must a Curlew, Plover, or Snipe, excepting that you have no other Sauce but Salt.

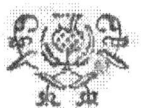

Directions *for trussing of* Fowls, &c.

How to truss a Rabbet for Roasting.

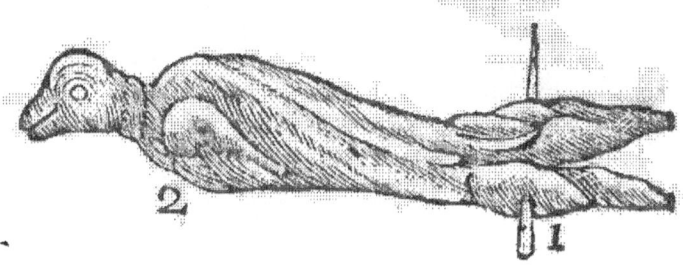

Explanation.

Case the whole Rabbet, except the lower Joints of the Fore-Legs, and those you should chop off; then put a Skewer through the Middle of the Haunches, after you have laid them flat, as at 1, and the Fore-Legs, which are called the Wings, must be turned as at 2, so that the smaller Joint may be pushed into the Body, through the Ribs. This is a single Rabbet, has the Spit put through the Head and Body, but the Skewer takes hold of the Spit to preserve the Haunches. But if you truss a Couple of Rabbets, there should be seven Skewers, and then the Spit passes through between the Skewers without touching the Rabbets.

N. B. You may truss it short, in the same Manner as for boiling, and roast it.

How to truss a Rabbet for boiling

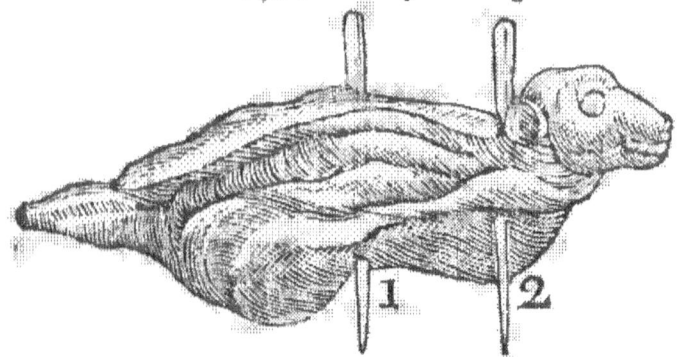

Explanation.

First cut the two Haunches close to the Back-bone two Inches, then turn up the Haunches by the Side of the Rabbet, and skewer them through the Middle of the Back, as at 1, then pass a Skewer through the Shoulder-Blades and Neck, and the utmost Joints of the Legs, as at 2. Bend the Neck backwards, and truss the Shoulders high, that the Skewer may be easily put through the Whole.

How to truss a Hare.

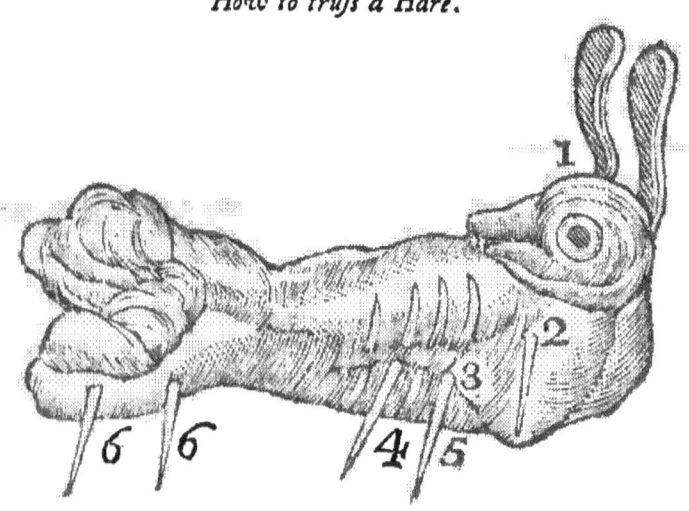

Explanation.

In cafing a Hare, when you come to the Ears, put a Skewer juft between the Head and the Skin, and raife it up by Degrees till both the Ears are ftripped, and take off the reft as ufual. Then twift the Head over the Back, as at 1, and put two Skewers in the Ears to make them ftand almoft upright, and to keep the Head in a proper Pofition; then pufh up the Joint of the Shoulder-blade towards the Back, and put a Skewer between the Joints through the bottom Jaw, to keep it fteady, as at 2, and another Skewer through the lower Branch of the Leg and through the Ribs, as at 3, to keep the Plate-bone up tight, and another through the Point of the fame Branch, as at 4; then bend both Legs in between the Haunches fo as to make their Points meet under the Scut, and take care to fkewer them faft with two Skewers, as at 6 6.

A Hare may alfo be truffed fhort, in the Manner of a Rabbet for boiling.

How to trufs a Pigeon.

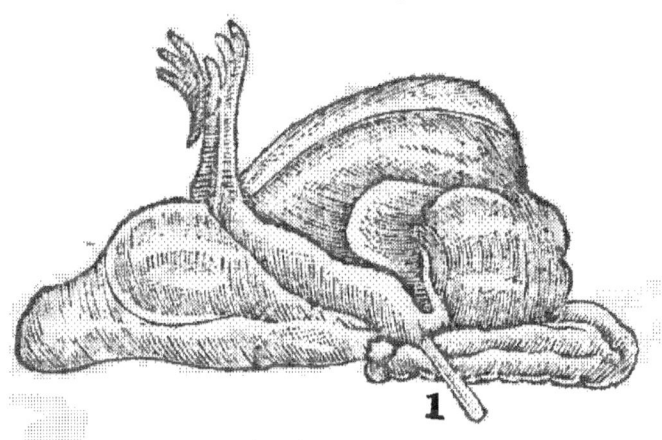

Explanation.

When you draw a Pigeon, leave in the Liver becaufe
it

it has no Gall; then pufh up the Breaſt from the Vent, and holding up the Legs, paſs a Skewer juſt between the Brown of the Leg and Bent of the Thigh, having firſt turned the Pinions under the Back; and take care that the lower Joint of the large Pinions are paſſed with the Skewer in ſuch a Manner that the Legs are between them and the Body, as at 1, and then you are right.

How to truſs a Fowl for boiling.

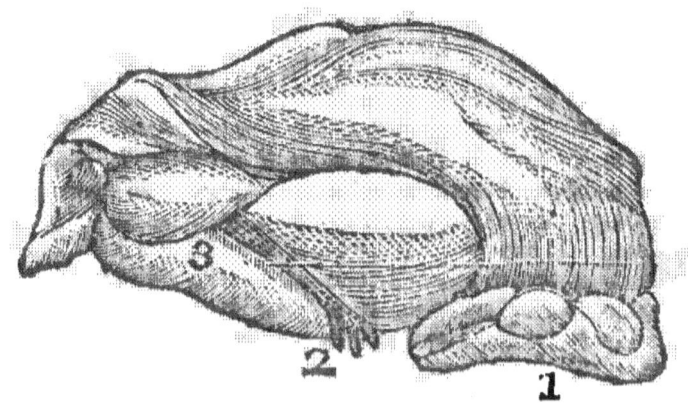

Explanation.

When you have drawn your Fowl, twiſt the Wings till you bring the Pinions under the Back, and thoſe who chuſe it may put the Gizzard and Liver, one in each Wing, as at 1, but they are generally left out. Beat down the Breaſt-bone to prevent its riſing above the fleſhy Part; then cut off the Claws of the Feet, twiſt the Legs, and bring them towards the Wing on the Out-ſide of the Thigh, as at 2, and cut a Hole on each Side of the Apron juſt above the Sideſman, and put the Joints of the Legs into the Body, as at 3, no Skewer being made uſe of.

The Young Woman's best Companion. 143

How to truss a Goose.

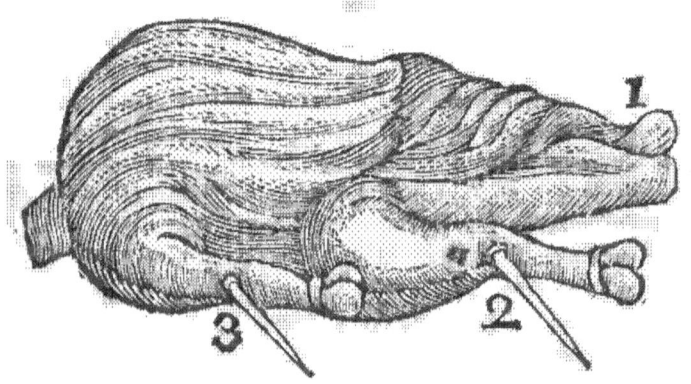

Explanation.

Let only the thick Joints of the Legs and Wings be left to the Body; the Pinions and the Feet should be cut off and go with the other Giblets, which consist of the Gizzard and Liver, and the Head and Neck. Cut a Hole at the Bottom of the Apron of the Goose, as at 1, and draw the Rump through it; then put a Skewer through the small Part of the Leg, and through the Body near the Back, as at 2, and another through the thinnest Part of the Wings, and through the Body near the Back, as at 3, and you have done.

How to truss Easterlings, Ducks, Teals, and Widgeons.

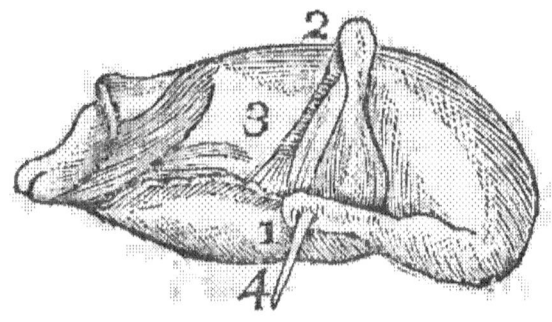

Explanation.

When you draw it lay aside the Gizzard and Liver, and take out the Neck, taking care to leave the Skin of the Neck full enough to cover that Part where the Neck was cut off. Next cut off the Pinions, as at 1, and raise up the whole Legs till they are in the Middle, as at 2, and press them between the Body of the Fowl and the Stump of the Wings; then twist the Feet, and bring the Bottom of them towards the Body of the Fowl, as at 3; and put a Skewer through the Fowl between the lower Joint, next the Thigh and the Foot, taking hold of the Ends of the Stumps of the Wings, as at 1, then the Legs will stand upright, and the Point of the Skewer will be at 4.

How to truss a Partridge or Pheasant.

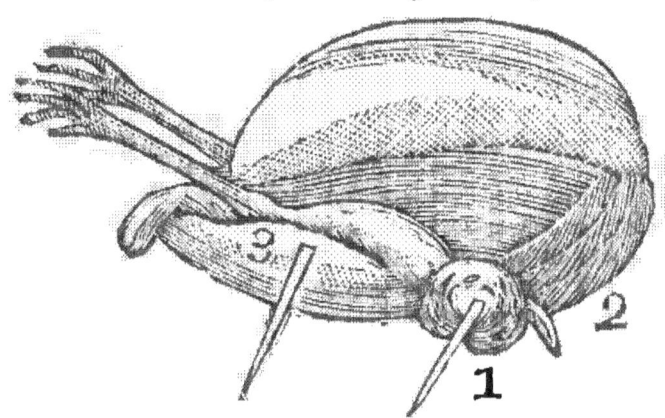

Explanation.

The only Difference between trussing a Partridge and a Pheasant is, that the Neck of the Partridge is cut off, and the Head of the Pheasant is left on. The above Cut represents a Pheasant trussed.

After having drawn it, cut off the Pinions, and leave only the Stump-bone next the Breast, then put a Skewer through its Point, and through the Body near the Back,

giving

giving the Neck a Turn; and paſſing it by the Back, force the Head on the Out-ſide of the other Wing-bones, as at 1, and put the Skewer through both; with the Head ſtanding towards the Neck, or the Rump, which you chuſe. The Neck ſhould go as at 2; then take the Legs and preſs them by the Joints together, ſo as to paſs the lower Part of the Breaſt; and then preſs them down between the Sideſmen, and put a Skewer thro' all, as at 5, and you have done.

A BILL *of* FARE *for every Month in the Year.*

JANUARY.

Firſt Courſe.

SOUPS of Peaſe, Gravy, Herbs, Fiſh, Vermicelli, &c.

Fiſh; as, Biſque of Fiſh, Carp, Soles, or Tench ſtewed, Turbot, Flounders, Plaiſe, Cod, Thornback, or Scate boiled, &c. Whitings broiled or boiled.

Bacon or pickled Pork, and Fowls and Greens in one Diſh.

Calf's-Head, or Knuckle or Veal, Bacon and Greens.

Collar of Brawn.

Leg of Pork boiled with Turnips, and Peaſe Pudding.

Leg of Lamb and Spinage.

Briſket of Beef ſtewed.

Ache-Bone or Rump of Beef, either boiled with Greens, or roaſted, with Horſe-radiſh, &c.

Turkey and Chine.

Neat's Tongue and Udder.

Pullets roaſted and Eggs.

Veal roaſted, ragou'd, boiled, &c.

Paſtry; as, Puddings and Pyes of various Sorts, Pancakes, Fritters, and minc'd Pyes.

Scots Collops

Broccoli, Aſparagus, Spinage, Cabbage-Sprouts, Coleworts, Cabbage, Savoys, Red and White Beets, Carrots, Potatoes, Horſe-Radiſh, Onions, Parſnips, Turnips, Leeks, Thyme, Sage, Parſley, Celery, Endive, Winter-Savoury, &c. are Gardenden-stuff to be had in this Month, as well as in the succeeding Spring Months.

Second Course.

Poultry; as, Wild Fowl of all Sorts, Turkey, or Chickens, roasted, with Asparagus.

Fish; as, Jowl of Sturgeon, Marinated Fish.

Roast Beef with Greens, or Horse-Radish.

Quarter of Lamb.

Hare roasted, with a Pudding.

Chine of Mutton roasted, with Pickles.

Pig roasted or collar'd.

Calf's Head or Hog's Head roasted.

Dry'd Tongues.

Pastry; as, butter'd Apple-Pyes hot, Lamb, and other Pyes.

Fruits of all Sorts; or Sweetmeats.

FEBRUARY.

First Course.

Soups of different Sorts.

Poultry; as Hen, or Turkey, with Oyster-sauce, or Eggs.

Fish; as, Cod's Head, &c. boiled; Tench, Carp, &c. stewed; Pike roasted, with a Pudding in its Belly; Whitings, Plaise, Flounders, boil'd or broil'd; Eels spitchcock'd, broil'd or boil'd.

Salt-Fish and Eggs, or Parsnips.

Salmagundy.

Scots Collops.

Ham and Chickens, with Sprouts or Broccoli, Lupines, &c.

Beef Marrow-bones, and black Puddings.

Chine of Mutton and Caper-sauce.

Second Course.

Poultry; as, Chickens and Asparagus, roasted Partridges or Quails, Squab Pigeons, young Rabbets roasted or fricasy'd; Turkey.

Fish; as, Soles, Flounders, Lobsters, Sturgeon, &c.

Pastry; as, Tarts, Cheesecakes, Pear-pye and Cream, hot butter'd Apple-pye, &c.

Sweetmeats.

Fruits of all Sorts.

MARCH.

MARCH

First Course.

Soup of Gravy, Herbs, Fish, Peafe, &c.

Fish of all Sorts, either fryed, broiled, stewed, or boiled; as Carp, Tench, Mullets, &c.

Neat's Tongue and Udder, with Greens, Roots, &c.

Stewed Veal.

Knuckle of Veal boiled, with Greens.

Ham and Chickens, or Pigeons.

Ache-bone or Buttock of Beef, with Greens and Roots.

Ache-bone, Rump, Sir-loin, or Ribs of Beef roasted, with Pickles, Horse-radish, &c.

Pastry; as, Marrow-puddings, Hogs-puddings, Almond-puddings, Battalia, and other Pyes.

Second Course.

Poultry; as, Chickens and Afparagus, Knots, Ruffs, Reeves, Ducklings, or Quails.

Fish; as, broiled Pike, Salmagundy.

Pastry; as, Skerret-pye, Tongue sliced with Butter, Pear-Tarts, with Cream, Jellies of all Sorts, Puffs of Apples, Marrow-puddings, Yolks of Eggs, &c. *Shrewsbury*-cakes, &c.

Fruits of all Sorts; as Apples, Pears, *China* Oranges, dry'd Grapes, *French* Plums, Almonds, Raifins, in this as in the two preceding Months.

APRIL.

First Course.

Poultry; as, Bifque of Pigeons, Rabbets or Chickens fricafy'd.

Fish; as, Mackarel, with Goofeberry-fauce, if to be had; Carp, Tench, &c. ftew'd or boil'd.

Beef boiled, roafted, or ftew'd.

Calf's-Head or Knuckle of Veal, or Fowls with Bacon and Greens, as Broccoli, Spinage, &c.

Neck of Veal boiled, with Rice.

Ham and Chickens or Pigeons, with Broccoli, or other Greens.

Chine of Veal, or Leg of Lamb, with Spinage, boiled or stewed.
Scots Collops.
Pastry; as, Lumber-pye, Veal or Lamb-pye, &c.

Second Course.

Poultry; as, Green Geese, Ducklings roasted, or sucking Rabbets, Chickens, and Asparagus.
Fish; as, butter'd Sea-crabs, fry'd Smelts, roasted Lobsters, Lobsters & Prawns, Crab-fish, Marinated Fish, pickled Salmon or Herrings, and sous'd Mullets.
Roast Lamb, with Cucumbers, or *French* Beans, if to be had.
Pastry; as, hot butter'd Apple-pye, Tarts, Cheesecakes, Custards, Rock of Snow, and Syllabubs.
Fruit of all Sorts; as, Nonpareils, Pearmains, Russet pippins, Bonchretien-pears, &c. Cherries and Raspberries, if to be had.

MAY.

First Course.

Poultry; as, roasted Fowls fors'd.

Fish; as, Jowl of Salmon boil'd with Smelts, &c. Carp and Tench stew'd; collar'd Eel, with Crayfish, &c. roasted Lobsters, Bisque of Shellfish.
Boil'd Beef, Mutton, Veal, with Greens, Roots, &c
Calf's-Head
Breast of Veal ragou'd.
Chine of Mutton with Pickles
Neat's Tongue and Udder, roasted or boil'd, with Colliflower or Broccoli, if to be had.
Beans and Bacon.
Pastry; as, Boil'd Puddings of several Sorts, Chicken or other Pyes.

Second Course.

Venison; as, Haunch of Venison, Leverets or Fawn roasted, Quarter of Kid, &c.
Poultry; as, Turkey-pouts, Quails, young Ducks, or Green Geese, roasted.
Fish; as, collar'd Eels, roasted Lobsters, Prawns, or Cray-fish.
Asparagus upon Toasts.
Green Pease.
Pastry; as, Orangado-pye, Tarts,

The Young Woman's best Companion. 149

Tarts, Cuſtards, Cheeſe-cakes, Creams, &c.
Fruits; as, Apples, Strawberries, Cherries, &c.

JUNE.

Firſt Courſe.

Veniſon; as, Haunch roaſted or boiled, with Colliflower, *French* Beans, &c.
Poultry; as, Fricaſee of Chickens, or young Rabbets; boil'd Pigeons with Bacon and Greens.
Fiſh; as Turbot, ſtew'd Carp, Tench, Soles, boil'd Trouts, Mullets, Mackarel, Salmon, roaſted Pike, or Barbels.
Lamb and Mutton, with Colliflowers, Cabbages, Kidney-beans, &c.
Beans and Bacon.
Breaſt of Veal ragou'd.
Ragou of Lamb-ſtones and Sweetbreads.
Weſtphalia or *Yorkſhire* Ham, with young Fowls.
Beef and Colliflowers.
Roaſted Pig.
Paſtry; as Marrow-pudding, Veniſon-paſty, Umble-pye, &c.

Second Courſe.

Veniſon; as, roaſted Fawn, Leverets.
Poultry; as, Pheaſants or Turkey Pouts, young Ducks, young Rabbets, Quails, &c.
Fiſh; as, Lobſters, Prawns, or Cray-fiſh, Jowl of Sturgeon, Fry of ſpitchcock'd or collar'd Eels, Chine of Salmon, butter'd Crabs.
Peaſe or Skirrets.
Paſtry; as, Potatoe-pye, Tarts, Cuſtards, Cheeſecakes, Creams, Jellies, Syllabubs.
Fruits of all Sorts; as, Cherries, Raſpberries, Strawberries, Gennetin Apples, and Pears, ſome early Figs, Currants, early Apricots.

JULY.

Firſt Courſe.

Veniſon; as, Haunch roaſted or boiled.
Poultry; as, Pigeons, Fowls, Bacon, &c. Green Geeſe.
Fiſh; as Freſh Salmon boil'd, Carp and Tench ſtewed, Mackarel, Turbot, Trouts boil'd, with butter'd Lobſters.

O 3 Beans

Beans and Bacon.
Calf's Head, with Bacon and Greens, or Colliflowers.
Scots Collops.
Chine of Veal.
Pig, larded.
Beef, or Mutton, boil'd or roasted.
Ham and Chickens, with Colliflowers, Cabbage, &c.
Roasted Geese, or Ducklings.
Pastry; as, Pigeon Pye, Puddings of several Sorts; Patty Royal, &c. Venison Pasty.

Second Course.

Venison; as, The Shoulder roasted; Potted Venison, in Slices; Hare, roasted.
Game and *Poultry*; as, young Ducks, tame or wild Partridges, Quails, Pheasant Pouts, Turkey Pouts, Pigeons, Rabbits, &c.
Fish; as, Soused Mackarel, Lobsters, or Prawns, Marinated Fish.
Potted Beef in Slices.
Collar'd Beef in Slices.
Pease.
Pastry; as, Tansy, Tarts, Custards, Cheese-cakes, Jellies.

Fruit; as, Pine Apples, Plums, early Grapes, early Peaches, and Apricots, Currants, Gooseberries, Rasberries, some Strawberries, Apples, Pears, Cherries, Filberts.

AUGUST.

First Course.

Venison; as, Haunch boiled with Colliflowers, Cabbages, or *French* Beans, or roasted, with Gravy and Claret Sauce.
Poultry; as, Fricasy of Chickens or Rabbets, forc'd Fowls, or Fowls *a la Daube*; Rabbets and Onions, roasted Turkeys larded, Geese.
Fish; as, Tench or Carp stew'd, Bisque of Fish.
Pig roasted.
Beef *a-la-mode*.
Beans and Bacon.
Chine of Mutton, with Pickles, or *French* Beans, or stew'd Cucumbers.
Ham and Chickens.
Pastry; as, Pigeon-pye, Umble-pye, Venison Pasty, Florendines.

Second

Second Course.

Poultry; as, **Turkey Pouts**, **Pheasants**, or **Partridges**, roasted **Chickens**, young **Ducks**.
Fish; as, **Lobsters**, roasted or cold, butter'd **Crabs** in Shells, or on **Toasts**, broil'd **Pike**, spitchcock'd **Eel**, collar'd **Eel**, **Salmagundy**, **Marinated-Fish**.
Calf's-Liver, or **Ox-Heart**, stuffed and roasted, with Gravy-Sauce.
Pork Griskins.
Collar'd Pig.
Potted Venison, in Slices.
Collar'd Beef in *ditto*.
Pease.
Pastry; as, **Tansey**, **Tarts**, **Jellies**, **Creams**, **Sweet-Meats**, **Rock of Snow**, and **Syllabubs**.
Fruits; as, **Melons**, **Grapes**, **Apples**, **Pears**, **Figs**, **Mulberries**, **Raspberries**, **Currants**, **Peaches**, **Apricots**, &c.

SEPTEMBER.

First Course.

Venison; as, the **Haunch**, &c.
Poultry; as, roasted **Geese**, **Pigeons** and **Bacon** boiled, **Rabbets** and **Onions**, **Pullets** and **Oysters**, with **Bacon**.
Fish; as, **Skate** or **Thornback**, **Bisque** of **Fish**.
Boil'd **Beef**, and Garden-stuff.
Leg of **Pork** with **Greens**.
Knuckle of **Veal**, **Bacon** and **Greens**.
Chine of **Mutton**, with a Sallad and Eggs.
Boil'd Leg of **Mutton** with **Turnips**.
Calf's Head and **Bacon**.
Pastry; as **Pigeon**, or **Squab-pye**, **Pork-pye**, a Pye with **Rabbets**, and **Pork Steaks**, **Lumber-pye**, **Venison-pasty**, **Beef-Stake Pye**, **Pork-pye**, with **Potatoes** cut in Dice, **Veal-pye**, **Battalia-pye**.

Second Course.

Poultry; as, **Ducks**, **Partridges**, **Pheasants**, **Teals**, **Pigeons**, roasted.
Fish; as, spitchcock'd **Eel**, fry'd **Smelts** and **Soles**, Jowl of **Sturgeon**, pickled **Salmon**, collar'd **Eel**, **Lobsters**.
Roasted Shoulder of **Mutton**.

Col-

Collar'd Beef in Slices.
Collar'd Pig, in *ditto*.
Cold Neats Tongue, in *ditto*, with Butter.
Peafe.
Artichokes.
Paſtry; as, hot butter'd Apple-pye, Cheefe Cakes, Tarts, Cream, Jellies.
Fruit; as, Melons, Apples, Pears, Figs, Peaches, Nectarins, Morello Cherries, Currants, Grapes, Mulberries, &c. Walnuts, Filberts.

OCTOBER.

First Courſe.

Veniſon; as, Haunch of Doe, boil'd with Garden-ſtuff.
Poultry; as, Bifque of Pigeons, Geefe roafted, Turkey with Oyfters.
Fiſh; as, Cod's-Head, with Shrimps and Oyfter-Sauce, Tench or Carp ftew'd, Gurnets.
Ham and Fowls, with Roots and Greens.
Bacon or pickled Pork and Fowls, or Pigeons with *ditto*.
Turkey and Chine.
Chine of Veal and Roots.
Chine of Mutton and Pickles.
Powder'd Beef, with Roots and Greens.
Scots Collops.
Pork falted and boil'd with Greens, &c. and a Peafe Pudding.
Paſtry; as, Lumber-Pye, Venifon Pafty, Mutton-pye, Pigeon-pye.

Second Courſe.

Poultry; as, wild Ducks, Teal, Wigeons, Eafterlings, Woodcocks, Snipes, Larks upon Skewers, Partridges, and Pheafants.
Fiſh; as, Eels boil'd, Smelts fry'd, Chine of Salmon broil'd or fry'd, with Anchovies and Shrimp-Sauce.
Salmagundy.
Artichokes.
Slic'd Tongue and Pickles.
Paſtry; as, Tarts, Cuftards, Cheefe-cakes, Jellies, Creams, Quince-pye, &c.
Fruit; as, Apples, Pears, Peaches, Nectarins, Figs, Plums, Grapes, Mulberries, Walnuts, &c.

NO-

NOVEMBER.

First Course.

Stew'd Beef in Soup, or good Broth.
Poultry; as, Turkey boil'd with Garden-stuff, roasted Geese, Hen Turkey roasted, with Oyster-Sauce, Rabbets and Onions.
Fish; as, Tench or Carp stew'd, Dish of Gurnets, scollop'd Oysters, and stew'd Carp.
Boil'd Leg of Pork, with Turnips and Greens.
Boil'd Haunch of Doe Venison, with Herbs and Roots.
Leg of Mutton boil'd, with Greens, &c.
Boil'd Fowls and Bacon, or Ham, or pickled Pork and Greens.
Chine of Mutton roasted, and Pickles.
Chine of Veal, with Pickles.
Breast of Mutton ragoo'd.
Ragoo'd Veal.
Calf's Head boil'd, grill'd or hash'd.
Ox-Cheek stew'd or bak'd.
Pastry; as, Venison pasty, Mince'd-pye, &c.

Second Course.

Poultry; as, Woodcocks, Snipes and Larks, Partridges, Pheasants, wild Ducks, Wigeons, and Teal.
Fish; as, Smelts fry'd, Chine of Salmon *ditto*, Marinated Fish.
Neat's Tongue, in Slices, with Pickles.
Collar'd Beef, in *ditto*.
Potted Beef, potted Hare, potted Pigeons, &c.
Pastry; as, hot butter'd Apple-pye, Pear-pye, with Cream, Potatoe-pye, Quince-pye, Jellies, Tarts, Cheese-cakes.
Fruits; as, Apples, Pears, Walnuts, Chesnuts, dry'd Plums, Grapes, &c.

DECEMBER.

First Course.

Soups of Gravy or Pease; or Plumb-pottage.
Poultry; as, boil'd Pullets and Oyster Sauce, or with Sausages, Rabbets and Onions, Hare grigg'd, Pigeons and Bacon.
Fish; as, Cod's-head with Shrimp

Shrimp and Oyster-sauce, and garnish'd with Smelts or Gudgeons, stew'd Carp or Tench, with Eels spitchcock'd or fry'd, stew'd Soles, Turbot, &c. Oysters before Dinner.

Ham and Fowls, boil'd with Greens.

Buttock of Beef, *ditto*.

Leg of Pork. Greens, and Pease-pudding.

Haunch of Venison boil'd, and Garden-stuff.

Leg of Mutton boil'd, with Turnips and Greens.

Leg of Lamb with Spinage, and the Loin fry'd in Chops, round the Dish.

Chine of Pork and Turkey.

Calf's Head and Bacon.

Sir-Loin of Beef roasted, with Colliflowers, Horseradish, &c.

Chine of Mutton and Pickles.

Pastry; as, Minc'd-pye, Lumber-pye, Veal-pye, Squab-pye, Venison-pasty, Battalia-pye, Marrow-puddings, &c.

Second Course.

Poultry; as, Capons, Rabbets, Hares, Turkeys, Pheasants, Partridges, Woodcocks, Easterlings, Snipes, Larks, Wild Ducks, Teal, Wigeons, Bustard, Squab-pigeons, roasted.

Fish; as, potted Lamprey, potted Chars, potted Eels, Jowl of Sturgeon, Lobsters, Bisque of Shellfish, &c.

Brawn in thin Slices.

Fore Quarter of Lamb roasted, and Mint-sauce, and Sallets, garnish'd with Orange.

Leg of ditto, boiled with Spinage, Loin in Steaks, round the Dish, and Orange in Slices.

Pastry; as, Tansey, Pear-Tart cream'd, potted Venison, Apple-pye, Tarts, and Cheese-cakes.

Fruits; as, China Oranges, Chesnuts, Pomgranates, Apples, Pears, dryed Grapes, &c.

Messes *for* Suppers.

Brawn, Ham, *Dutch,* or Hung Beef.
Collar'd Beef, Mutton, Pig, Veal, Pork, Eel, &c.
Potted Beef, Pigeons, Hare, Venison, Eel, Char, Lampreys, Trouts, &c.
Neat's Tongues, Calves, Stags, or Sheeps Tongues.
Stew'd Beef, Veal, Mutton, Hare, Pigeons, Ducks, wild Fowl, Pig.
Ox or Calf's Heart stuff'd and roasted; Sheep's Heart.
Hash'd Veal, Mutton, Beef, or Lamb, with Pickles.
Minc'd Veal, &c.
Mutton or Beef, Sweetbreads and Kidnies.
Veal Sweetbreads ragou'd.
Lamb's Liver and Bacon fry'd.
Hog's Liver, Crow, and Sweetbread fry'd.
Calf's Liver and Bacon fry'd, or roasted and stuff'd.
Tripe fry'd, boil'd, or fricaseed.
Eggs and Bacon.
Eggs in Shells.
Eggs poach'd.
Eggs poach'd, and Spinage stew'd.
Salmagundy
Sallets of different Sorts, according to the Season.
Pig Pettitoes.
Beef Steaks and Oysters, or with Gravy and Horse-Radish, or with a Relish of Anchovy, or Walnut Pickle.
Scots Collops.
Veal Cutlets.
Mutton Cutlets, or Chops, with Pickles or Horse-Radish, or with Sauce made of Capers, Butter, and a little Sugar.
Chickens boil'd with Parsley and Butter, or roasted.
Rabbets fricasee'd, or roasted.
Butter'd Turnips.
Artichokes.
Potatoes.
Anchovies, Walnuts, Cucum-

cumbers, and other Pickles.
Pickled Herrings, Oysters, Salmon, Sturgeon, &c.
Mackarel boil'd, sous'd, or broil'd.
Cod and Oyster Sauce, Trout, Soles, Smelts, Gudgeons, Tench, Carp, Whitings, Skate, Plaise, Flounders, &c. Lobsters, Crabs, Prawns, Cray-Fish, Oysters, and other Fish in Season.
Tarts, Cheese-cakes, Custards, Jellies, Sweet-meats, Pyes, Pasties, and Fruits according to the Season.

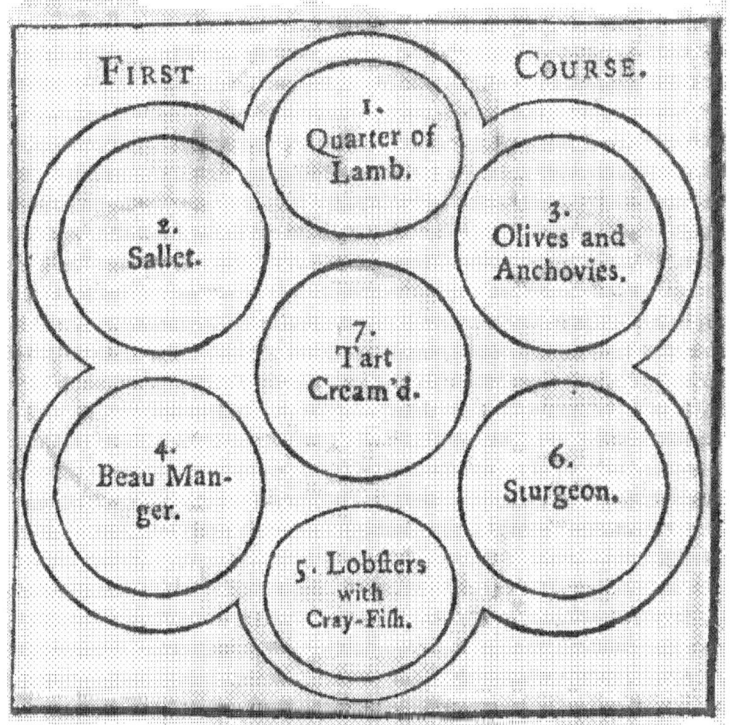

1 Cold Chickens.
2 Tongue.
3 Pickled Salmon.
4 Tarts of several **Sorts**.
5 Stew'd Pippins.
6 Prawns.
7 Olives.

1 Cold Beef.
2 Sallet.
3 Potted Lobsters.
4 Ice Creams.
5 Cray-fish.
6 Custard-pudding.
7 Smelts.

158   *The Young Woman's best Companion.*

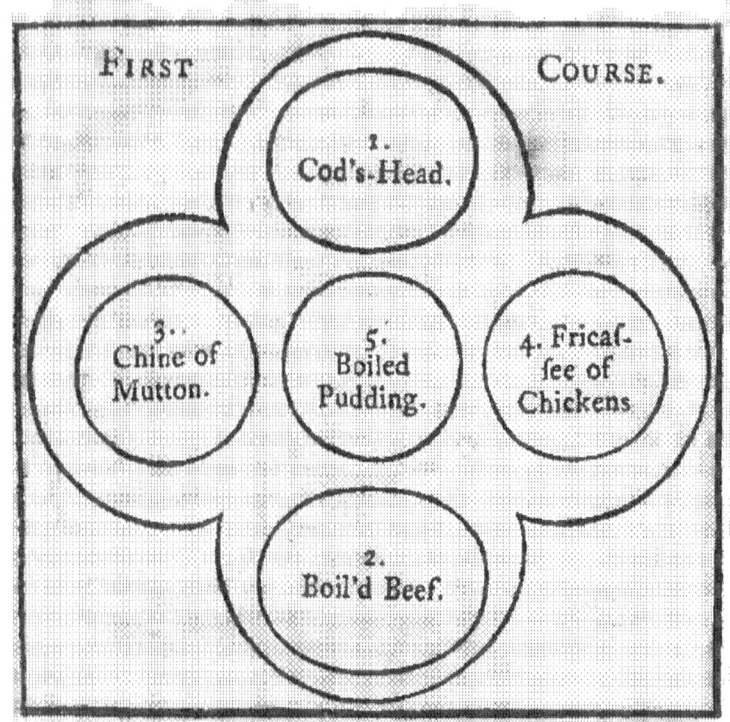

Second Course.

1 Ducklings.
2 Roasted Lobsters.
3 Pigeons and Asparagus.
4 Cray-fish.
5 Crocand.

First Course.

1 Chickens.
2 Ham.

3 Stew'd Tench.
4 Quarter of Lamb.
5 Tansey with Fritters.

Second Course.

1 Green Goose.
2 Venison.
3 Prawns.
4 Olives, &c.
5 Pear pye.

FIRST

The Young Woman's best Companion.

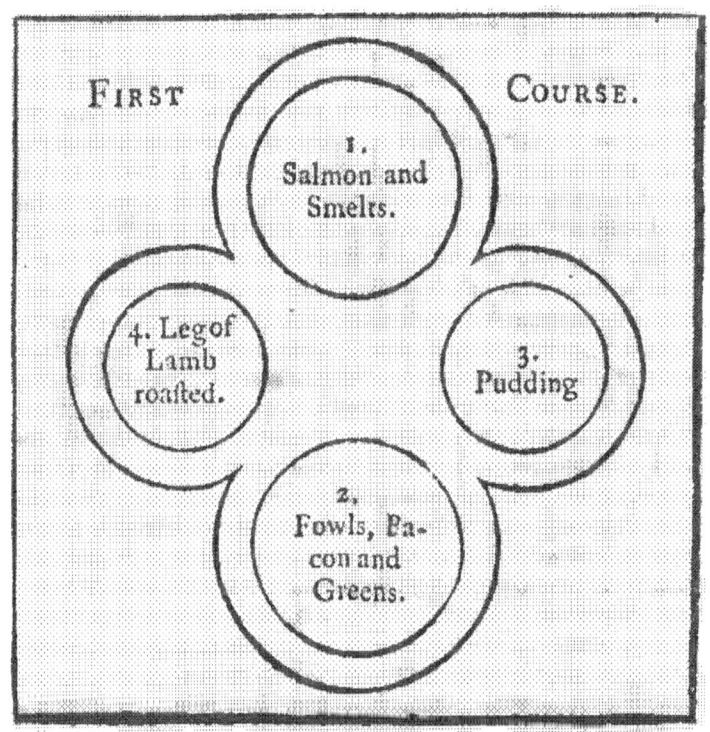

FIRST COURSE.
1. Salmon and Smelts.
4. Leg of Lamb roasted.
3. Pudding
2. Fowls, Bacon and Greens.

Second Course.

1 Ducklings.
2 Roasted Lobsters.
3 Tansey.
4 Sweetbreads.

First Course.

1 Boiled Beef.
2 Fillet of Veal.
3 Palpatune.
4 Fry'd Soles.

Second Course.

1 Hare.
2 Fricasee of Chickens.
3 Cray-fish.
4 Blomange.

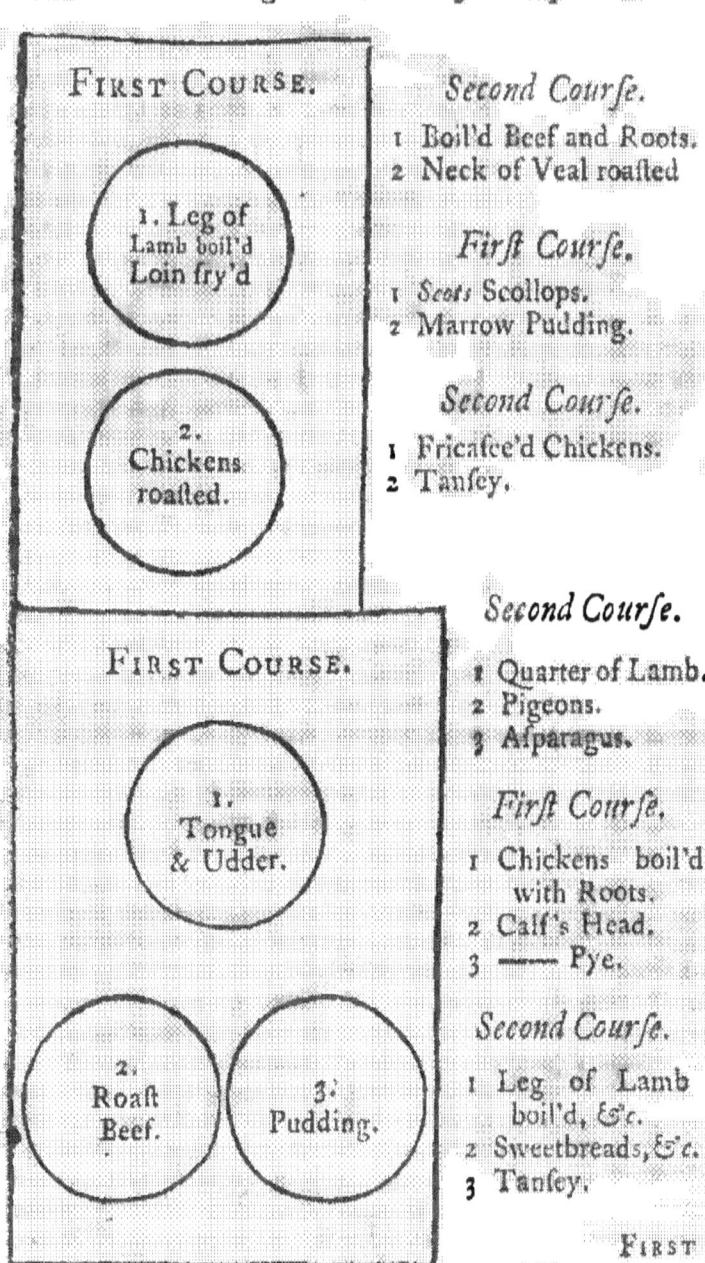

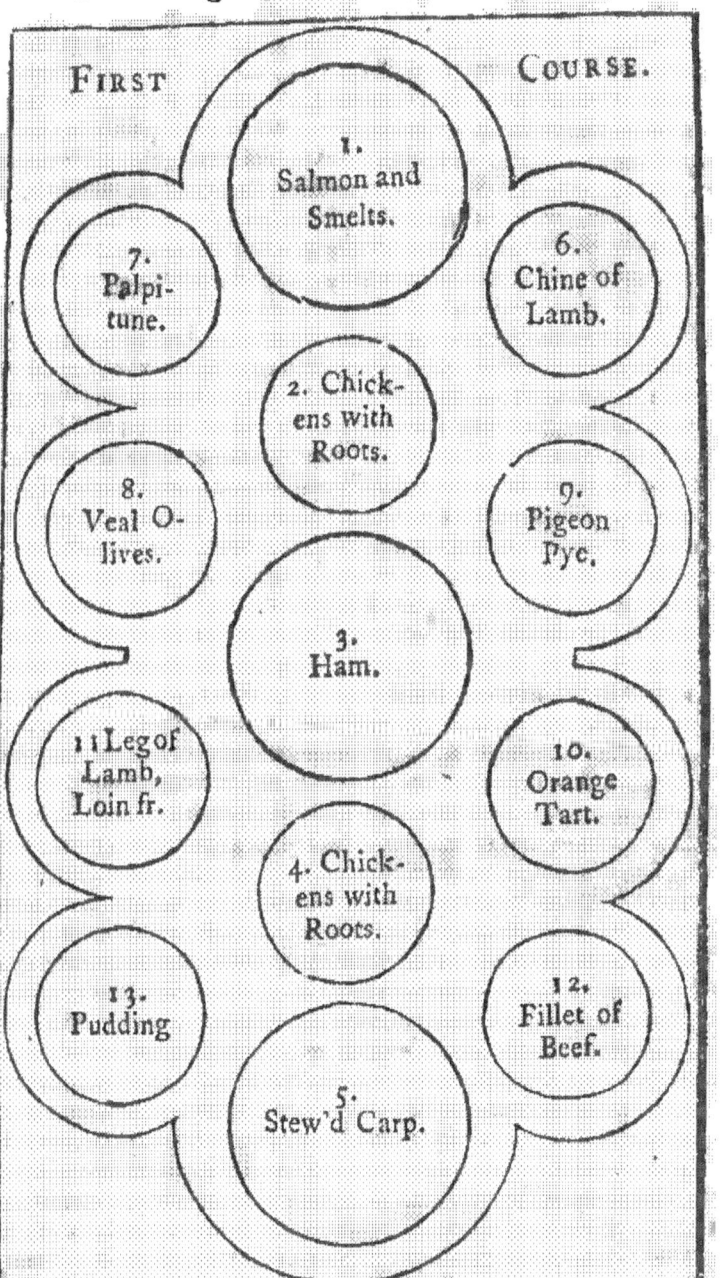

Second Course.

1. A Green Goose.
2. Lobsters.
3. Crocand.
4. Sturgeon.
5. Two Ducklings.
6. Asparagus.
7. Sweetbreads.
8. Snipes.
9. Tansey.
10. Olives, &c.
11. Prawns.
12. Blomage.
13. Potted Wild Fowl.

Another First Course.

1. Soup Remove, with Fish.
2. Chickens with Bacon and Roots.
3. Roast Beef.
4. Chickens with Bacon and Roots.
5. Fish and Soup.
6. Potted Wild Fowls.
7. Veal Olives.
8. Marrow Pudding.
9. Chickens a la daube.
10. Ragoo of Mushrooms.
11. Quails.
12. Cray-fish
13. Stew'd Pippins.

Second Course.

1. A Green Goose.
2. Sweetbreads.
3. Asparagus.
4. Lobsters
5. Woodcocks.
6. Tansey.
7. Crocand.
8. Prawns.
9. Olives, &c.
10. Sturgeon.
11. Potted Wild Fowl.
12. Blomage.
13. Ducklings.

Course for Dinner.

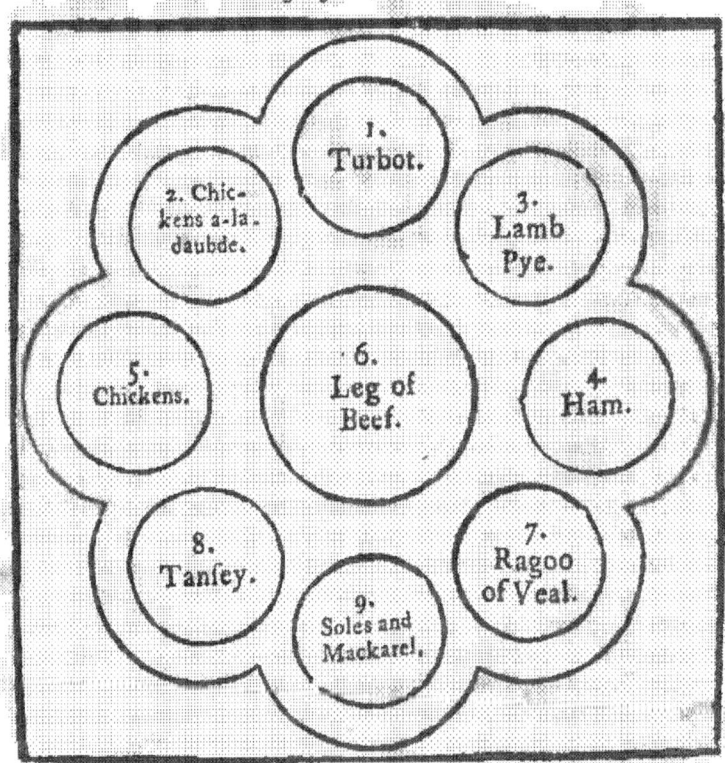

Another.
1 Soup Remove, Ham and Chickens.
2 Snipes or Woodcocks.
3 Pheasants or Fowls roasted.
4 Bread-pudding.
5 Fricasee of Lamb, Chickens, or Rabbets.
6 Pigeon-pye.
7 Fry'd Soles or Cray-fish.
8 Chickens boil'd with Colliflowers.
9 Sir-Loin of Beef.

FINIS.

THE CONTENTS.

	Page	to	Page.
Directions for Marketing, from	1	to	7
for all Sorts of *Fish*	7	to	10
The Weight and Sizes of the Loaves of Bread, made by the Authority of the Magistrates	11		
The proper Seasons for all Sorts of Provisions	11	to	12
Instructions for dressing all Sorts of common Provisions	12	to	18
Directions concerning Poultry	18	to	20
General Directions for Boiling	20	to	24
Instructions for boiling of all Sorts of Greens	24	to	29
for dressing of all Sorts of Fish	29	to	38
for broiling, frying, basting, stewing and baking all Kinds of Meat	38	to	51
Directions for making of all Sorts of Fricassees	51	to	53
General Rules to be observed in making of Soups or Broths	53	to	58
in Potting and Collaring	59	to	66
Instructions for making Puddings, Dumplings, Pancakes, and Fritters of all Sorts	66	to	74
Rules for making all Sorts of Meat-Pies	74	to	83
Instructions for making all Sorts of Fruit-Pies, Tarts, Cheesecakes, and Custards	83	to	90
Instructions for making various Kinds of Cakes, Gingerbread, Biscuits, Macaroons, Wigs, and Buns	90	to	96
Instructions for making Cream Jellies, Syllabubs	96	to	104
divers Sorts of Jellies	105	to	107
Pickling and Preserving	107	to	115
The British Vintner; or Rules for making all Sorts of Fruit Wines	116	to	121
The Compleat Brewer; or Directions for brewing all Sorts of Beer and Ale	121	to	125
The Family Physician and Dispensatory	125	to	136
Instructions for Carving	136	to	138
for trussing all Sorts of Fowls, &c.	139	to	145
A Bill of Fare for every Month in the Year	145	to	156
Directions for placing Dishes	157	to	163

www.ingramcontent.com/pod-product-compliance
Lightning Source LLC
Chambersburg PA
CBHW022117160426
43197CB00009B/1068